HEALING *through* CHRONIC PAIN

A Physical Therapist's
Personal Journey
of Body/Mind/Spirit
Transformation

MARY RUTH VELICKI, MS, DPT

D1167056

Alley Press
Los Angeles, CA

HEALING THROUGH CHRONIC PAIN
Copyright © 2013 by Mary Ruth Velicki

Printed in the United States of America.

Alley Press, Los Angeles, CA
ISBN-13: 978-1490966618
ISBN-10: 1490966617

Library of Congress Cataloging-in-Publication Data
Velicki, Mary Ruth
Healing through chronic pain: a physical therapist's personal journey of body/
mind/spirit transformation / Mary Ruth Velicki
ISBN-13: 978-1490966618
Library of Congress Control Number: 2013912661

First edition published by Alley Press, 2013

Cover and interior design by Ana C. R. Magno, Los Angeles, CA

www.healingthroughchronicpain.com

For my husband,
Alex,
and my children,
Katherine and Alex III,
for standing beside me in the dark
and for teaching me about life and love

Acknowledgements

I am incredibly grateful for my team of caregivers who compassionately pushed me down the healing road. One of the main reasons I began writing was to share their helpful wisdom, and now their knowledge, advice, and encouragement fill these pages.

My team of caregivers, in order of appearance on this journey are: Michelle Ryan, MD; Stuart Chalfin, MD; Jacqueline Gray, PhD; Stella Tryon, Registered Yoga Teacher (RYT) and Reiki Master Teacher (RMT); Julie Sarton, Doctor of Physical Therapy (DPT) and Women's Health Clinical Specialist (WCS); Karen Noblett, MD; Pam Jacobsen, Licensed Acupuncturist (LAc) and Diplomat of Oriental Medicine (DiplOM); Mika Bursch, Licensed Massage Therapist (LMT); Chris Hernandez, Certified Massage Therapist (CMT) and RMT; Iben Larssen, RMT; Nicole Vasquez, DPT and WCS; Cris Law, Doctorate of Musical Arts (DMA) in progress; and Karen Axelrod, CMT and Diplomate-Certified CranioSacral Therapist (CST-D).

I greatly appreciate all those who generously read earlier versions of this book and provided much-needed encouragement and guidance: Karen Axelrod, Chris Hernandez, Andrea Kunihiro, Jeff Kunze, Richard Laliberte, Iben Larssen, Christine Nichols, Lee Sianez, Katherine Velicki, and the writer's group at the Unitarian Universalist Church of Long Beach, California.

Heartfelt thanks to Ana Magno for creating the cover design and interior layout of this book and to Colleen Sell for her careful editing. Colleen's experience and talent were especially crucial in bringing this book to life.

Contents

Preface

In 2007, I was moving through my life like a passenger on a high-speed train, always rushing toward a new goal and rarely stopping to enjoy the scenery flying past me. Then, suddenly, pain reared up in the very core of me and hurled me right off that train! I landed with an excruciating thud and watched the train cars roar past me like a bullet toward the orange horizon. As I lay writhing in the dust, I looked around and found myself surrounded by a dark desert without another soul in sight.

Not one to sit for long, I scrambled up and tried to walk, but the pain had turned into a huge backpack that made it difficult to move. Before, I had always charged through life looking over my shoulder at the past or peering up the road into my future. Now, the heavy weight of pain stooped me over so I could see only the ground directly beneath me. Before, I had run down all sorts of paths, driven by nagging neediness and fueled by incessant inner dialogue. Now, I moved more slowly. I had energy only for my most crucial tasks, and side trips were out of the question. Before, I had prided myself on being an independent, capable walker. Now, I often collapsed into an exhausted heap by the side of the road. Sometimes when I was lying in the dust, another soul would see me and haul me back onto my feet. Some of these helpers had familiar faces, and others were complete strangers. Once in a while, the person had special advice or skills that helped ease my pain and lighten the load on my back.

Sitting by myself in the dark, I often pulled the pack toward me and peered inside. I could easily see the physical pain, but over time I also started to see the mental and emotional pain that were intertwined with the physical discomfort. For more than five years, I walked down many different avenues trying to rid myself of the relentless pain. In my quiet moments, I studied the interior of that pack trying to identify the psychological factors contributing to my painful burden. When I found old issues, habits, fears, and beliefs that were weighing me down, I gently lifted them out and laid them at the side of the road.

Slowly, almost imperceptibly, the pack lightened over the years, and I began to hear the individual voices of my body, mind, and spirit. The path became increasingly clear and opened up before me, and I often just stopped to feel the glow of the sun on my cheeks or to gaze at the moon and stars. I noticed others walking beside me, too, and I felt a loving kinship with these strangers, friends, babies, and animals. In time, I realized I was walking through my life in a totally new way, and I made a conscious decision to keep walking that path rather than re-board that fast train. That is when it also occurred to me that the pain and suffering I had cursed for wreaking havoc in my life had actually been a catalyst for positive transformation in my life.

The road I'm traveling still has bumps and turns, and sometimes my pack feels a bit heavy again. But now, instead of spinning in fear, I usually just take a deep breath and experience all of it, because I know that even the difficult moments are a valuable part of the journey.

Introduction
Memos from the Fire

"The human being is a surprisingly resilient organism. We are impelled toward health not sickness. Your spirit, as surely as your body, will try to heal. . . . So you should not fear tragedy and suffering. Like love, they make you more a part of the human family. From them can come your greatest creativity. They are the fire that burns you pure."
— Kent Nerburn, *Simple Truths: Clear and Gentle Guidance on the Big Issues in Life*

Before chronic pelvic pain threw me off-track at age forty-five, I was busy and productive, and ideas about spirituality and the mind-body-spirit connection never really entered my mind. But when the pain took hold and wouldn't let go, I was forced to step out of my life for more than five years to pursue all sorts of healing avenues and to look deeply within. Much to my surprise, the suffering was actually a gift. It opened up an opportunity for growth and led to deep healing at all levels of my person. Don't get me wrong; it was the most difficult challenge of my life so far, and I needed tremendous help in my healing process. But comparing my life and the state of my body, mind, and spirit before my illness to now, I would never want to go back. The journey was rocky, but the rewards were unexpected and amazing.

At the very beginning of my illness, I began writing a guide on how to physically manage chronic pelvic pain. Having a reason for going through the pain made it easier to endure, and writing was a natural extension of my career as a physical therapist and university instructor. But then this journey became about much more than just relieving my physical pain and writing a book to help others manage their chronic pain. Unexpectedly, this intense experience woke up the spiritual side of me. I also discovered many tangible connections between my body, mind, and spirit—which would have seemed implausible for my scientific, Western-medicine–trained mind just a few years before. As I grew, the perspective of the book expanded, too. Because I wrote during the struggle itself, rather than summarizing the experience at its end, these pages capture the changes that took place in my whole being throughout the five-year healing process.

The first section of this book describes the challenges and changes that occurred at all levels of my person (social self, body, mind, spirit) during the first two years of intense pain as well as the direct connections I experienced between the different aspects of my being. The second section of this book chronicles the last three years of my illness, when I was actively working to uncover what I was carrying at deeper emotional and spiritual levels that might be contributing to my pain. The process of looking within led to deep healing of my whole person. I landed more firmly into my authentic self, and both my internal and external life began to transform.

For me, the catalyst for positive personal change was chronic, intense pelvic pain. For you, the catalyst may be another form of chronic physical pain, or psychological pain, or some other struggle. When I first started sharing the stories I've included in this book with friends, neighbors, and even strangers, it surprised me that people who had not experienced chronic physical pain could also relate to my journey. But I soon realized that painful struggle and transformation are deeply human experiences and that much of what I experienced on an individual level is also universal. Although different catalysts may start the process, transformation often involves the same unfolding of the layers of body, mind, and spirit and the same gradual healing through these layers.

Before my illness, I worked as a physical therapist specializing in the treatment of people who had suffered neurological injuries, such as stroke, brain injury, and spinal injury. It was a blessing to stand beside these people during such an intense time in their lives. Sometimes, my patients were in despair; sometimes, they were digging deep to find meaning and hope. Throughout the experience, I felt connected to them through our shared humanness and vulnerability.

When I've told my story to other people and shared with them the advice and encouragement I've received along the way, I've seen their faces light up with recognition and felt a similar loving connection between us. This feeling of being connected with other people at a deeply human level was crucial for my own healing, and I suspect the same is true for others. I wrote this book with the hope that my experiences will provide connection, support, and guidance to others on their own healing journeys.

For Readers with Chronic Pain

During the peak of my pain just a few months into my illness, I was curled up in bed reading the book *A Headache in the Pelvis*, by David Wise, PhD, and Rodney Anderson, MD. When I got to the part where a physician talked about his suffering with pelvic pain, I exclaimed loudly, "I know exactly how you feel!" In that moment, I felt less isolated and lonely, and when I read that this doctor had improved over time, I also felt some hope. My friend Christine, who beat stage-three breast cancer, told me that she was always on the lookout for stories of people who had good outcomes. She wrote them down or cut them out, then stored them in her "Hope File." These stories helped get her through when she thought she would never get better. If you are on a difficult leg of your journey, file my story under "hope."

Before I would even start reading someone else's story, I'd want to know, *Did he or she get better?* So I'll answer that question right off the bat: Yes! I did get better. And in this book you will find the advice and methods that helped me to heal physically. As I worked through the pain, I realized that some of my skills as a physical therapist and teacher enabled me to look at my condition in an analytical way and to communicate effectively with members of my care team. In order to get better, I pursued a wide variety of healing avenues from Western, Eastern, and alternative medicines, and I was incredibly fortunate to work with a group of very experienced and skilled professionals. One of the biggest reasons I felt compelled to write this book was to share their helpful wisdom with others who are in pain.

Keep in mind that there are many different medical issues, underlying theories, and treatments for chronic pain, and the combination of these will be different for every person. The process I went through to heal my body is unique to me and presented as an example for others to consider; it is not a prescription for everyone with chronic pain. Please discuss your individual case with your own caregivers.

In this book, the term "caregivers" refers to anyone providing care, such as physicians, therapists, and holistic health practitioners. Although my pain is centered in the pelvic region, the information in this book may be helpful for others with different chronic pain conditions, especially those that are also multi-factorial and complicated, like fibromyalgia.

Early in my illness, I was most aligned with my analytical mind, so I started on this journey *thinking* my way through the pain—but later I learned to also *feel* my way through it. Over time, I realized that my illness created challenges and changes for my mind and spirit as well as for my body. I came to understand that all three aspects of my person—body, mind, and spirit—are interconnected pieces of this healing puzzle. Taking this holistic approach to my illness ultimately played an integral role in my healing, so I decided to write about all aspects of my experience.

When my pain was new and intense, I found a book online with a title that was something like One Woman's Spiritual Journey with Interstitial Cystitis. The exact title eludes me because I didn't read the book. I thought, *Who cares about her inner experience. I just need my body to get better.* If this is where you are, you may want to begin reading the sections in this book that describe the concrete steps I took to relieve my physical pain (especially Chapter 3 and the appendices).

As I was finishing this book, a little mental image popped into my head that seemed to summarize what you are about to read. At first, we will stroll and talk around the edges of a pool, but eventually, I will take your hand and plunge into the deep end. The whole experience is here, and you can decide whether you want to ramble in the sunshine, swim in the depths, or jump in and bob quickly back to the surface!

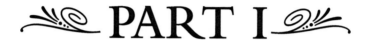

PART I

My Pain,
My Catalyst for Healing

*"In the depth of winter, I finally learned that there was
within me an invincible summer."*
— Albert Camus

1

Pain Explodes and Healing Begins

In the summer of 2007, I spent my days taking care of our home, driving my two teenagers (ages thirteen and fifteen) to their activities, and working as a physical therapist. My professional duties included teaching an Internet course, treating a private patient, and taking a course at the local university. During my leisure time, I enjoyed working out, shopping, and watching television with my kids.

My life was busy, but I was often alone and lonely. My main social contacts were with my husband of nineteen years and my children. Even though I visited with people at school events, in my neighborhood, and at the gym, I didn't have any close friends.

Before the onset of my pelvic pain, I was aware of only a couple of my internal struggles. One struggle I was conscious of was my concern that I would no longer be able to work as a physical therapist because staying current in my treatment skills was important for teaching. Throughout my career as a physical therapist, I had specialized in neurological rehabilitation. Working with these patients was physically demanding, and I was concerned my body was no longer up to the challenge due to aging and past injuries. In addition, I was aware of the hurt and frustration I felt about the lack of connection with my extended family, all of whom lived across the country from me. My mother had died five years before the onset of my illness, I had little contact with my siblings, and my father seemed to be giving up on life.

Still, life was rolling along fairly normally and comfortably, in much the same way as it had for years. . . . But everything was about to change.

Just Make It to Rome

One Monday in August 2007, a week before our long-awaited bus tour of Europe, I went to see Dr. Ryan, my internal medicine and general practitioner (GP). Over the weekend, I'd had a sudden onset of abdominal cramping and diarrhea that had quickly passed, but I thought I should get it checked out before the trip.

Dr. Ryan entered the room with a big hello. In her late forties at the time, Dr. Ryan was no-nonsense, experienced, and smart. She always asked about my family and me, carefully listening and remembering all the details that accumulated over the years. I mentioned to her that over the past few months the urge to urinate had been more intense and I had to make more trips to the bathroom. This was new. I didn't have a history of urinary tract problems, with the exception of cystitis (bladder inflammation) for a couple of months when I was in my twenties. Dr. Ryan found blood in my urine, a common sign of infection, and prescribed an antibiotic (Cipro®).

Instead of feeling better, however, a pain ignited in the center of my lower abdomen. The pain was both throbbing and sharp, and it intensified over the next few days. It felt like my bladder was extremely full and someone was sitting on my stomach. I went back to see Dr. Ryan, and she changed the antibiotic (to Macrodantin®). As I was leaving, I asked her if I could get the bladder anesthetic Pyridium® in case the discomfort continued during my trip. She didn't think I'd need it, but she prescribed it to ease my mind. On Thursday, I called Dr. Ryan again because the pain was worse, and she added another antibiotic to my regimen (Keflex®).

On Sunday, the day before we were to leave for our trip, I was still hurting. I called Dr. Ryan, but because it was her day off, I reached the female doctor who was on call. Partway through our conversation, she told me I sounded really anxious.

Perturbed by her comment, I responded, "Of course, I feel anxious. I'm leaving for Europe tomorrow, and after a week of treatment, I am getting progressively worse rather than better."

She then suggested I reconsider going on the trip because the rigors of a European tour can be difficult even when one feels healthy. She told me I was on all the right medications and maybe the pain was the result of another condition, like interstitial cystitis (IC), rather than infection. I knew from my medical background that IC referred to chronic inflammation of the bladder.

"I've heard that can be really painful," I said.

"Yes, it can," she replied.

I knew the doctor could do nothing more for me, so I quickly got off the phone. I was just enduring and hoping my symptoms would subside over the next day. On a conscious level, I didn't let in the possibility that I may have interstitial cystitis, but I suspect hearing those words set off some deep internal alarms. My anxiety continued to escalate.

My husband, Alex, seemed oblivious to my discomfort. When I told him I was in pain and was unsure whether I should go on the trip, he told me it was too late to cancel and that he and the kids were going with or without me. He said it wouldn't be nearly as fun if I didn't join them, but we had already paid for the trip. The thought of being by myself for two weeks seemed so daunting, isolating, and lonely. I didn't want to be left behind, and I didn't know what to do.

That night, for probably the first time in my life, I couldn't sleep and paced for hours in the dark. In addition to the pain, my hands were cold and shaky, and I felt a tingling sensation that started at the base of my neck and ran down my spine. At four in the morning, I thought, *Maybe this is related to anxiety.* I drank a full cup of wine, took a long hot shower, and breathed deeply. The pain lessened, and I decided to go on the trip.

One hour into the flight, the pain rose to the point where I was doing deep breathing to calm myself. I looked over at Alex as he sat reading quietly across the aisle. Although we were both in our mid-forties, he still looked the same to me as on the night we'd met when I was twenty-two. His classic features, five-o'clock shadow, brown eyes, and tall, lean build were so familiar, they gave me some comfort.

Four hours later as the plane began its descent into Atlanta, I reached over, tapped Alex on the arm, and said with resolve, "The pain is just too much. When we land, I'm going to fly back home instead of taking the connection to Rome."

But a few moments later, we ran into thunderstorms, which diverted the flight and delayed landing. We missed our connection, and Alex rebooked our flights to Europe for the following day. I was relieved to have more time to make my decision. That night in the hotel room while lounging on the bed eating pizza with my kids, I felt fine and decided to make the trip.

The next morning the pain was back, and I called Dr. Ryan from the hotel room. I was hoping she would prescribe a different medication that I could pick up at a local pharmacy on our way to the airport. Instead, she told me I needed to finish the antibiotics and be off of them a full week before she could do anything else. Meanwhile, she suggested I take Motrin® around the clock to decrease the bladder spasms. Whether I spent the next two weeks at home or with my family in Europe, she said, was up to me.

Alex reassured me. "Just make it to Rome. If you feel bad, I'll fly you home. If you feel really bad, the whole family will go home with you. There are airports in all the major cities, and if you need to, I can get you home."

Although wary and anxious, I also believed him. So I decided to head to Europe with the family.

I made it through our two-week European tour with two antibiotics, Motrin, and Pyridium on board. I often caught Alex studying me from across the bus or the room, and he frequently stood beside me while we listened to our guide and whispered, "How are you doing?" It was much easier to endure the discomfort with his support. Over those two weeks, the intensity and duration of the bladder pain gradually decreased. Sometimes when the bladder pain subsided, I could feel a pulling and tightness anywhere from my pubic bone to the coccyx (tail bone). Whenever the pain would lift, it felt like I was stepping out of a fog to be awed by the sights around me.

On our last day in London, however, new symptoms cropped up. My chest became tight, and I felt shaky. Nevertheless, I still walked for miles in the drizzly rain, determined to take in those last sights.

Then, on the eighteen-hour flight home, my fever rose to 102 degrees Fahrenheit. I went directly from the airport to Dr. Ryan's office. She told me I had the flu and asthmatic bronchitis, and prescribed antibiotics and an inhaler. She was concerned that my bladder pain had persisted throughout the vacation, especially since the urine culture taken before the trip showed no signs of bacteria. She ordered another urine culture and a pelvic ultrasound and referred me to a urologist, Dr. Chalfin.

Adding Grief to Physical Pain

The phone was ringing when I returned home from my appointment with Dr. Ryan. The call was from my sister-in-law, who lived across the country in the same town as my father. She told me they'd found my dad unconscious on the floor of his living room that morning. The CAT scan showed a huge bleed on his brain, and the prognosis was not good. I called Dr. Ryan and asked if I could fly to Chicago to see my dad, but she said my lungs were too bad to make the flight. My dad never regained consciousness. He had brain surgery the next day and died later that week.

During that time, the flu and bronchitis resolved. But the bladder pain returned, and my hands once again became cold, clammy, and shaky. My body was constantly calling for my attention, and it didn't even register with me that my father was gone.

Before I flew to the funeral, I met with the urologist, Dr. Chalfin. He sat across from me and patiently listened as I went through my history and list of questions. He told me that the recent urine culture and pelvic ultrasound showed no signs of pathology, but there was still blood in my urine. He encouraged me to try meditation and yoga to calm down my nervous system.

Five days later, the pain level was still high, so Dr. Chalfin performed a cystoscopy, inserting a flexible tube with a lighted tip up my urethra and into my bladder, which enabled him to look at the interior lining of those areas. He told me the bladder was inflamed. He then performed an internal pelvic exam and palpated my pelvic-floor muscles. He noted that I had a muscle spasm deep on the left side with a knot as big and hard as a marble. He prescribed the muscle relaxant Vesicare® to decrease the spasms in my bladder and put me on a diet that I later found out was commonly recommended for people with IC. Dr. Chalfin had a theory that strengthening the muscles of the pelvic floor would decrease the bladder spasms and pain, so he showed me some exercises for that purpose, called Kegels.

The pain was so intense I had to fight to keep my concentration while I shopped for funeral clothes for myself and my family, wrote my father's obituary, and flew to Chicago. Before my father's wake, I went alone to his casket and studied his handsome, boyish face and his thick, agile hands, even though every detail was already firmly planted in my memory. When I touched his face, it was hard and cold; only then did it register that he was gone. It felt like déjà vu. I'd had the exact same experience five years before when my mother passed away.

I stood beside my dad's body for hours, greeting lines of relatives, neighbors, friends of my parents, and parents of my friends. How bittersweet it was to see all these people I held in my heart but who lived so far away. Although I'd moved to California twenty-three years earlier, parts of my mind and heart still resided in my hometown.

The next day as I watched my dad's casket being lowered into the earth alongside my mom's, my only thought was, *There is no more time to connect.* I would understand later how this sense of disconnection in my life was intricately wrapped up in my pain.

Diagnosis and Fear

I had been through a lot during the month of August, and my doctors thought I just needed time to calm down and heal. Instead, the pain continued throughout the month of September, and my anxiety steadily escalated.

Even though I was hurting, I kept up with my exercise routine. In mid-September as I was climbing the StairMaster© next to Carolyn, who is a physician, I told her about my fears of having a chronic pain condition. She suggested I see a therapist to talk about my feelings and to decrease some of the emotional burden on my husband. Shielding my family made sense to me, so I called Dr. Ryan, and she referred me to a psychologist.

Then, Dr. Ryan said, "The cystoscopy report says possible beginning stages of interstitial cystitis."

"Dr. Chalfin never mentioned that diagnosis to me," I replied.

Dr. Ryan apologized and then read the full report to me.

Later that week, I called Dr. Chalfin's office to make a follow-up appointment. The receptionist asked me if I knew my diagnosis. I told her I hadn't been told directly, but my family doctor had informed me of Dr. Chalfin's report citing possible interstitial cystitis. Her voice dropped and sounded full of dread when she said, "I just wanted to see if you knew."

I didn't tell anyone that the term "interstitial cystitis" had already been screaming in my head for two weeks and I'd been thinking of little else. My mind was spinning to the worst-case scenario. I kept replaying a scene from a radiology class I had taken several years before. The professor had shown the class a radiograph of a woman's bladder that presented obvious signs of calcification and stated that the woman had interstitial cystitis. He told the class he felt so badly for the poor women who came to his office with this diagnosis because they would be in such pain and they would try everything, but nothing ever worked. Some even tried having surgery to remove the bladder, but the nervous system was still intact, so the pain remained. For some women, the pain was so great they had committed suicide.

I distinctly remember sitting in that classroom and thinking, *That might be me.* This thought seemed really random, because I had no bladder symptoms at the time. But I remember everything about that moment: the location of my professor, my position in the classroom, the picture on the screen, even how my body felt sitting in my chair.

After Dr. Ryan told me I might have interstitial cystitis, I went online and read a few medical articles about the condition. I quickly jumped to the worst-case scenario. I envisioned myself going to the bathroom every fifteen minutes day and night, suffering horrible bladder pain, and becoming totally isolated. I thought, *The life I've known has ended, and any happiness I can glean from this point on is just extra.*

My pain was getting worse, so I made another appointment with Dr. Chalfin. Toward the end of my visit, I mustered up the courage to ask, "Do I have interstitial cystitis?"

The doctor was seated across the room, facing me. He looked down and then to the right before replying. "I don't give that diagnosis lightly." That was all he said, but he prescribed Elmiron®, which I knew was the only medication approved for IC. He also suggested I sit in a warm bath to decrease the pain and again encouraged me to try yoga or meditation.

I remember quite a bit of what Dr. Chalfin said to me that day, including these words: "I am happy to hear that you are seeing a psychologist, because this condition doesn't get better unless you get the limbic system [a lower part of the brain involved in the processing of emotions] under control." . . . "You have a moderate case of this condition." . . . "Take it easy on yourself; you can't fix this with your mind." . . . "Come back to see me in a month."

As I was leaving the office, I thought, *How can I live with this pain for a month?*

Alone in the Dark

When I came home from Dr. Chalfin's office, I was terrified and completely alone. Alex was in Germany on a two-week business trip, and I didn't have a support network beyond him. I didn't tell Alex how badly I felt because there was nothing he could do from so far away and I knew he wouldn't come home unless it was an emergency. I also didn't want to appear needy because, before he left, Alex seemed frustrated by my escalating anxiety.

The two weeks Alex was away on business coincided with the darkest time of my illness. Dr. Chalfin encouraged me to rest, but I was in pain and in overdrive—taking the kids to athletic practices, back-to-school nights, and church; working out daily; and setting up eight additional activities and appointments. My bladder hurt all day and would not let me rest. The pain would often wake me from a deep sleep, and I would lay there frightened by how much it hurt. I couldn't eat, and in two weeks, I lost ten pounds.

Here is a journal entry from that time:

If this is my life, how can I possibly get through it? How many more years until the kids are raised, and how can I make it? If no one loved me, I could check out, but people are counting on me. I'm trying to be positive, trying to find meaning, trying to be grateful. I'm tired. The illness is hidden, even to myself. In the mirror, my face looks exhausted, lined, tear-stained, and pained. I feel like I'm trapped in my own personal hell. Can I give the pain to you for just a minute, so you can feel the cross I bear?

Adding Insult to Injury

I diligently performed my Kegel exercises, hoping that stronger pelvic-floor muscles would decrease the painful bladder spasms. When I wasn't getting better after several weeks of doing Kegels, Dr. Chalfin sent me to a physical therapist who used biofeedback and exercises to strengthen the pelvic-floor muscles. This treatment is traditionally used to help women with an overactive bladder and urinary incontinence, but Dr. Chalfin thought it was worth trying.

During the two weeks Alex was on his trip, I attended four appointments with this physical therapist. On my first appointment, she asked me to insert a sensor, which looked like a plastic tampon, into my vagina, and then she watched a monitor that displayed the level of activity in my pelvic-floor muscles. Instead of the diminished activity typically seen in patients with weak pelvic-floor muscles, the resting/baseline activity of my muscles was consistently high. Whenever I performed a Kegel exercise, the muscle activity would rise quickly and then sink very slowly toward this elevated baseline. After each exercise, the physical therapist would repeat, "Relax, relax, relax." It didn't matter how calm I tried to be, my muscles remained pulled up tight.

This therapist responded to my anxiety with lots of advice. She encouraged me to get on with my life, ignore the pain, and pretend everything was just fine. She told me that when she went out with her friends for dinner, she had to tell herself to not focus on her own knee pain and to have a good time.

I thought, *The pain is so bad I'm having trouble eating or sleeping. I can't even imagine going out to dinner with friends.*

She continued with her advice: "You need to get your mind over your bladder." . . . "The pain is just in your brain." . . . "There are different perceptions of pain in different cultures. Some women just squat, have a baby, and then keep on working.". . . "You are too negative; you need to write down a list of all the positive things in your life."

I should have shouted, "You have no idea of what I'm enduring! I'm a positive person who is really suffering!" Instead, I was polite and took it all in, but inside I was devastated.

At the end of my fourth treatment session, the therapist again told me I needed to be a more positive person—because, if I were depressed, no one would want to be around me. That comment sent me reeling, as my worst fear was to be abandoned in my suffering. I had been trying to handle the pain by myself, but I felt like I was sinking fast.

Unexpected Compassion

As soon as I got home from my fourth—and last—visit with that physical therapist, I walked across the street to my neighbor Lee's house and broke into tears. "I look normal, but I feel like a cat—barely holding on with my nails," I sobbed.

During the twenty years Lee and I had been neighbors, we'd often visited when we saw each other in our front yards and at occasional neighborhood events, but we didn't really socialize. Still, I'd always felt comfortable with Lee, who is fifteen years older than me and a warm and gregarious person, and at that moment, comfort was exactly what I needed. Even though Lee seemed surprised and a bit overwhelmed by my emotional outburst, she held me like a mother and wiped away my tears.

The next evening I was doing laundry in my garage when another long-time neighbor, Kelly, walked her dog in front of my house. She continued up my driveway and commented about how thin I was, and I went out to greet her. As I told her about my condition, concern flashed in her sparkly blue eyes. Although Kelly and I had always shared a mutual respect, we weren't close friends. From that moment on, though, she often walked down the street to quietly check on me.

The day after I broke down in Lee's arms, I had my first appointment with the psychologist to whom Dr. Ryan had referred me a few weeks earlier, Jacqueline Gray. When I told Jackie my history with the pain and started to sob, she expressed empathy for me. She told me her bladder had also been inflamed for a full year, and she described exactly how this particular pain grated intensely on your nerves.

"You are in too much pain," she said. Then she repeated my words from the day before, "You are like a cat—just barely holding on with your nails."

Jackie called Dr. Ryan to discuss possible pain medications. She gave me instructions in deep breathing and visualization, and told me to make an appointment to see Dr. Chalfin again.

As I was walking out the door, I confessed, "My husband, Alex, is so active that I worry he won't want to be around me if I can't keep up."

"Do you need to be perfect in order to be loved?" she replied.

Her comment hit home. For that and many other reasons, I knew Jackie was the right therapist for me.

By then it was early October, and Alex came home. I laid on the bed as he unpacked and told me about his adventures in Germany. When he said he was looking forward to going back to Europe with me, I told him I wasn't sure I would be able to travel again.

"You did it before; you can do it again," he said.

I started to cry and finally confessed to him what I had been going through while he was away. I explained how I'd wanted to handle everything alone and shield him from it, but the pain was just too big. I told him Jackie had said I couldn't protect him and this was part of his journey, too.

Alex hugged me and told me Jackie had given me good advice and I shouldn't worry about him. He said we would handle it together and protect the kids. As I lay there crying in his arms, I could feel the bladder pain lift a little bit.

The next day I had an appointment with Dr. Ryan. I told her, "I don't really feel depressed, but the pain is so great that I sometimes feel like a caged animal. It's like internal nerve pain, and it's even worse than when I hurt my neck and had all that pressure on the nerve root."

She looked at me with concern and compassion. She told me I was strong and stoic, and when I said my pain level was a level four, she knew most of her other patients would describe it as a level ten. She said I was the type of patient who could get into trouble because the pain level I report doesn't reflect how bad it is. She gave me a prescription for an antidepressant that is also used to decrease nerve pain (Cymbalta®).

That evening I was mentally fuzzy, but I also felt the pain melt away to a more manageable level. I knew the medication could take several weeks to work, so I suspected my relief was just a placebo effect. But I didn't care how it was working; I just knew the voice screaming "Interstitial cystitis!" was gone. Now that my mind was a bit quieter, I could appreciate how much I had been spinning with fear and anxiety. I thought, *If this is normal, where was I before?*

More Medical Drama

"This illness just keeps on giving!" I exclaimed to Alex one night.

In the second month of pain, I started to experience bouts of rapid intestinal voiding, also known as dumping and fecal urgency, which occasionally plagues people with pelvic pain. My first experience of dumping happened when I was four blocks from home on our nightly walk. Suddenly, I doubled over with major intestinal cramps and a feeling like someone was stabbing me in the rectum with a knife. I sat there writhing on the grass in someone's front yard as Alex ran to get the car. Thank goodness, he is a runner! I got to my home bathroom just as all the contents of my intestines made a beeline for the exit.

In addition to these occasional dumping incidents, I also started to have fecal urgency. In this case, I ran to the bathroom the minute I had the sensation of a possible impending bowel movement, because it was coming whether I got there or not. Fortunately, my pelvic muscles were so tense they could brace against a tsunami, so I never had an embarrassing accident.

At that point, the bladder pain was intense, relentless, and my most debilitating symptom. Every week, Dr. Chalfin's nurse performed an instillation in which the medication dimethyl sulfoxide (DMSO) was inserted directly into my bladder using a catheter. This medication is the only drug approved by the US Food and Drug Administration (FDA) for bladder instillations. It is not known exactly how DMSO works, but some patients experience pain relief, so it may block pain, decrease bladder muscle spasms, and/or decrease inflammation.

After my first DMSO instillation, I walked into the kitchen, and my husband and kids covered their noses and asked me to leave the room. I found out that a negative side effect of a DMSO instillation was that I would smell like garlic (or, as my kids reported, "burnt creamed corn") for about a day. I couldn't smell it, but others around me sure could! The clinicians hadn't told me about this side effect when I had the instillation, so I was glad I hadn't stopped by the store on the way home from Dr. Chalfin's office.

However, even after changing my diet, taking Elmiron for two months, and enduring eight weekly instillations and four physical therapy appointments, my pain was still intense for most of the day.

Building a Team

I asked to be referred to a different physical therapist, one who could perform manual work on my internal pelvic-floor muscles. I knew the muscle spasms in this area were not being addressed and were a big part of my problem. I didn't tell Dr. Chalfin that my visits to the first physical therapist had been completely destabilizing and that her take on my condition and advice were opposite to what Dr. Ryan and my psychologist were telling me. At that point in my care, I was too timid to speak my truth.

I now realize that even though the first physical therapist worked with women with pelvic issues such as incontinence, she did not have training in or knowledge of chronic pelvic pain. Dr. Chalfin told me that very few therapists have the extra training needed to work internally on the pelvic-floor muscles, and finding a physical therapist with that background can be difficult. I told him that I may be able to find someone through my professional contacts, and we agreed that each of us would search for a possible therapist.

On my next visit, Dr. Chalfin gave me a piece of paper with the name on it of the same physical therapist I'd found on the Internet the week before: Julie Sarton. Julie and I had already talked extensively on the phone, and I could tell by her line of questioning that she was very knowledgeable in the area of pelvic pain.

When I showed up for my first appointment with Julie, she strode toward me in her lab coat, smiling and with her hand outstretched. Her manner was professional and efficient, but her voice and touch were soft and compassionate. As physical therapists, we had many common experiences to draw upon, and she made me feel like I had known her forever.

I was impressed with Julie and surprised by the Women's Healthcare Center at the University of California (UC) Irvine where she worked. The urogynecologist leading the effort, Dr. Noblett, was respected, current, proactive, and experienced. I decided to transfer my care from Dr. Chalfin's office to this comprehensive center. The doctors, nurses, and physical therapists worked as a team, so communication was optimized and the multiple services I needed were coordinated.

Both Julie and Dr. Noblett recommended that I work with Pam Jacobsen, an acupuncturist who also specialized in pelvic pain. Prior to becoming an acupuncturist and opening her clinic, the Healing Sanctuary, Pam had been a registered nurse, which was comforting to me. Beyond providing skilled treatments, Pam saw me as a full person and guided me in alternative medicine options.

At the Healing Sanctuary—a calming atmosphere lit with candlelight and adorned with artwork—I met two other caregivers who were crucial for my healing. The first practitioner, Chris Hernandez, is a massage therapist and Reiki master who has experience working with women in pelvic pain. She joined my healing team eighteen months into my pain, and we worked together sporadically for about two years.

The second practitioner, Iben Larssen, is a Reiki master who has traveled the world for over two decades studying the diverse ways humans of different cultures have been healing themselves. Iben's practice combines energetic bodywork, like Reiki, with multi-dimensional life coaching that addresses state of the mind and emotions as well as the spirit and body.

We began working together two and a half years into my illness. We met consistently every week for a full year, and since then, I've seen Iben occasionally as issues surfaced.

In the fourth year of my illness, two other practitioners joined my care team: a new physical therapist, Nicole Vasquez, and Karen Axelrod, a massage therapist who is skilled in the alternative treatment, CranioSacral therapy.

Working with this group of women was a true blessing. Not only were they experienced and knowledgeable, they were also supportive and kind, which was healing, too. I will include myself in this healing group, because even though these amazing women provided me with skilled treatments and loving guidance, I had to make my own journey through the pain and toward my own healing.

Serendipity

At one of my acupuncture treatments, Pam brought up the concept of serendipity, a phenomenon in which something highly unlikely and beneficial happens seemingly by chance. This concept was interesting to me because, during the first two months of my illness, I experienced many such "fortunate occurrences," which made me shake my head and smile at the time. Following are a few examples.

On the day I met Jackie, my psychologist, she looked at me and said, "You are like a cat holding on with your nails." Those were the exact words I had used the day before to describe myself to my neighbor Lee!

Jackie was a good fit for me at the very beginning of my illness because she had suffered with the same type of bladder pain for a full year. Since she had personally felt this unique pain and experienced how it grated on her nerves and depleted her mental resources, she could give me the compassion, tools, and hope I needed to help me work through it.

My next lucky coincidence was finding Julie, my physical therapist, on the Internet and then having Dr. Chalfin hand me a piece of paper with her name on it. Julie was crucial to my recovery. Not only is she a pioneer in the use of physical therapy for chronic pelvic pain, but she also opened the door to a whole team of caregivers for me.

Finally, when Pam put in a request to my insurance for twelve visits of acupuncture, the returning authorization granted me one hundred visits. I needed, and used, every one of them.

The possibility of serendipity did not seem totally crazy to me because when my mom was failing, I had witnessed many happenings in her life that seemed to be more than just good luck. For seven years my mother struggled with amyotrophic lateral sclerosis (ALS), more commonly known as Lou Gehrig's disease. With ALS, the motor neurons progressively die, and without this communication between the brain and the muscles, the person gradually becomes paralyzed. I lived across the country from my mom, so we weren't together often. But on my brief visits to her home, I witnessed the following examples of serendipity.

On one visit I exited the limo from the airport, walked into my mother's home, and found her sitting in a chair at the kitchen table. After I put down my luggage and gave her a hug, I asked her how she was getting around. She said that once she was up, she could walk with the walker all around the house by herself. The problem was that she couldn't stand up from the chair by herself anymore. This was a new issue, and she hadn't told anyone but my dad about it.

The very next day, a friend brought her an electric elevating chair that had just been donated to the church and asked if she would be interested in it. Was she ever! She was once again independent.

On another visit I found her sitting in a wheelchair, just stuck in that one place. She could no longer walk or push the chair by herself. I called an equipment salesman to come to the house to meet with her, and he showed her pictures of electric wheelchairs. Her face lit up when he asked, "Would you like to move on your own?" However, for my frugal, Depression-era parents, coughing up approximately $10,000 for the chair plus even more money for a customized van in which to transport it was way too extravagant. They politely said they would think about it. As the salesman was leaving, he placed a brochure on their dining room table.

The next week at the ALS support group meeting, someone asked if any member were interested in buying a converted van with a lift for a ridiculously low price. My parents went to see it and decided to buy it. As they were leaving, the seller said, "I also have a nearly new wheelchair that I want to give you." He brought out a wheelchair that was the same exact model and color as the wheelchair in that brochure in their dining room.

My mom was almost giddy as she rode the chair around the neighborhood. Sometimes, she went so far that my dad had to take the car to find her!

My mother always said that when she needed nursing care, she wanted her good friend to be her nurse. Unfortunately, this friend already had a full-time nursing job and lived a half hour away. But right when my mom needed a nurse, her friend lost her job and became available for part-time work. And just when my mother's nursing-care needs increased and the commute became difficult for her friend, the friend decided to move to a smaller home. When she found her perfect house, it just happened to be three doors down from my mother's home!

When I was in pain, I would replay my mother's serendipitous experiences in my mind. It gave me faith that good things could happen to me, too, and it helped me to see my own moments of serendipity. Over the years, I also came to appreciate how complicated and powerful my relationship with my mother was. Some of our interactions were intricately wrapped up in my pain, and others gave me the hope and inspiration I needed to heal. This book is full of things I learned from my mother and from our relationship that helped me along this journey of body/mind/ spirit healing. This book is also filled with "positive coincidences" I have personally experienced that have helped me through this tremendous challenge in my life.

Signposts

During the first year of pain, I had an appointment with a different caregiver almost every day. They did not talk with each other about my case, so it was interesting that on some weeks they would all tell me the same thing from their unique perspectives. After the third or fourth time the same message came through, I knew I should perk up my ears and listen.

In addition, when I was working through something emotionally, the same message would often come to me from several different sources within a few days, and just to be sure I got it, the message often arrived in the same exact words. Often, complete strangers told me things that perfectly matched what I was working through at the time, and their words gave me a new perspective or validated the path I was on. About three years into my pain, my life coach, Iben, told me that when you reach a certain level of personal awareness, you start noticing that people can be like messengers in your life. This phenomenon would continue and even expand over the healing years.

These messages also came in the written word. Before my pelvic pain began, I rarely read for pleasure. But during this journey, a few books were given to me at a key time or were recommended by several people over a few days, and each was incredibly helpful.

Some of these helpful writings were my own, written about thirty years before my pain descended. I found my teenage journal about two years into my pain and was shocked to see that many of these writings clearly spelled out the pain and patterns of my life that I was currently working through.

Almost five years after my pain began, I found a few poems I had written for a class in college that were tucked away in the pages of my old journal. To my surprise, the poems depicted many of the core issues I had been working hard to uncover and move through in order to heal from my pelvic pain. Reading those poems, penned in my own young handwriting, validated my healing process and made me wonder whether I had always known my inner truth on some level.

All of those spoken and written words became signposts for me along the rough journey through chronic pain. They assured me I was traveling in the right direction and helped guide me through the next turn. They gave me hope that I was moving forward and that help would be provided along the way. Throughout this book, I share many of those messages—which always arrived right on time to show me the way out of the dark and move me down the road of healing.

2

Suffering Alters My Life and My Perspective

My personal focus and the healing throughout this journey seemed to move from outside to inside—from external issues to progressively deeper internal issues. So it makes sense that the first changes I experienced were related to my connection with the world, such as my work, my roles, and my relationships. During that time, the pain was quite a force, and its constant pressure changed my life and shifted my perspective during the first year or so of pain.

Everyday Heroics

When the pain began, I was still teaching a physical therapy class at Western University of Health Sciences. Although most of the course was online, I had to get through two weekends of live instruction. At the start of the first weekend, I walked into the classroom with my ego and expectations at an all-time low and thinking, *I'll just do my best today and hope it's okay*. I was different, and to my surprise, so were the students. Instead of generating competition and intensity, this class flowed back acceptance and kindness. They didn't know I was hurting, but it was one of the most loving classes I had ever taught.

On the second weekend session, one of the students asked me to join him for lunch. He was blind and grateful for the efforts I had made to accommodate his disability throughout the course.

"Thanks," I said, "but I'm having some discomfort today (huge understatement) and should probably rest during the break." I'd forgotten that to a physical therapist, the statement, "I'm having some discomfort," is a call to be questioned.

He was persistent, and finally, I told him about the pelvic pain. He asked if he could give me a therapy session after class, and he wouldn't take no for an answer.

So there I was, lying on the treatment table and pouring out my whole story as he lightly massaged specific acupressure points. At that point in my journey, allowing myself to be cared for and vulnerable was totally out of character and a testament to my desperation. I think it was easier to let down my guard because he was blind and couldn't see me.

I told him I had been surprised when Dr. Ryan, my internist and family doctor, had described me as strong and stoic. The student said he didn't see me as tough but rather as warm and compassionate. At the time, I didn't know myself very well and was always looking to others for my truth. This man didn't have the gift of physical sight but he sure had insight, and on that day, he saw my inner person more clearly than I did.

The whole weekend, I taught with a heating pad on my belly and a little Motrin in my system. While lecturing, I didn't feel the pain, but the minute there was a break in the material, the discomfort would rise up and I'd have to fight to stay focused.

After the last session, I went home and flopped on the couch. Alex brought me dinner.

"I can't believe I got through that," I said to him. "I feel like a rock star."

On my next visit with Dr. Ryan, I told her this story. As she left the examination room, she peeked around the door and said, "You *are* a rock star."

Honestly, when I was in pain, sometimes just getting through a regular day took heroic effort.

Where Is My Entourage?

At my father's funeral, soon after the onset of my illness, I told my sister, brothers, and sisters-in-law that I was in pain and worried about having a chronic condition. After months passed with no one having contacted me,

I wrote a letter to my siblings telling them about my diagnosis and what I had been experiencing. Another month went by, and with the exception of two calls from my sister-in-law, no one else contacted me.

During a counseling session, I read the letter to Jackie and we talked about it.

"Maybe I didn't make it clear what I was going through," I said.

She assured me the letter was very clear.

"Maybe my letter got lost in the mail," I said. "Or maybe they're traveling."

Looking at me with compassion, Jackie said, "I think you have a fantasy about this family."

The stress of difficult situations has a way of shedding light on the true nature of relationships, for better or worse. Many other people who had dealt with illness or loss warned me that the people I thought would be there for me may not show up and that the people who did support me wouldn't always be whom I expected. That certainly was true for me. Beyond my husband and children, all the people I thought were in my inner circle were not there when I got sick. I was very disappointed, hurt, and angry.

Jackie encouraged me to take off the rose-colored glasses and see my relationships for what they were. She assured me that if I lifted the illusion, I wouldn't be alone in the dark and would see light from other sources.

At one of my acupuncture visits, I told Pam I was confused by my family's lack of support, because I thought they loved me. She said they may love me but may not be strong enough to provide any support. She suggested that maybe they were absorbed in their own problems.

On our nightly walk, I told Alex what Pam had said.

"That makes sense," he replied. "Every engineer knows you can't put a load on something fragile."

The Loneliness Factor

During the second month of pain as I lay curled up in bed in the middle of the afternoon, too exhausted to do anything else, I noticed a book collecting dust on a nearby shelf: *Love and Survival: 8 Pathways to Intimacy and*

Health, written by cardiologist Dean Ornish. My friend Sandy had given it to me about a year before. Although I never read for pleasure, I picked up the book and started reading in an attempt to distract myself from the discomfort. When I came to Dr. Ornish's observation that people who get sick are often those who feel isolated, I gasped! That definitely fit my experience.

For me, this feeling of isolation had actually preceded the onset of pain—as expressed in the following passage from my old journal (which I discovered two years after the onset of my pelvic pain):

I'm lonely, lonely, lonely. I sit in a crowd of "friends" that pair off and become strangers. I'm pretending to have a good time, hoping that my smile will become authentic. I want desperately to be happy and to be close to people. I feel I have to entertain to get them to like me, to push to have them want to be near me, and to be lively to capture their applause. I'm tired of the chase.

These words, written at age nineteen, clearly described a feeling of disconnection that had not dissipated with age. Before the pain began, I was really busy—but also really lonely. I felt like I had few close relationships beyond Alex and the kids. A distinct thought came into my mind right before my pain began: *The only people I really talk to are those who perform services for me, like my doctor and hairdresser.* That underlying sense of disconnection loomed even larger after the pain began limiting my ability to work and to do activities that used to keep me so busy.

Every time Alex went out of town on business, my pain would always flare up. I also started to notice that when feelings of isolation would arise within me, the pain would often follow. When a caregiver would ask, "What do you think triggered the flare-up?" I would often respond, "The loneliness factor."

Let's Hear It for the Boys!

During the first few years of my struggle with chronic pain, my teen daughter, Katherine, seemed unaware of my illness and unaffected by the changes in our household. That was fine with me; I was grateful she was independently handling all the demands of her honors courses and running practices. Three years into my pain, when Katherine heard me describe my experiences to some family members, she was surprised that she'd had no idea of what I was going through at the time.

In the beginning, my husband and son were the ones in tune with me. They kept showing up, no matter how weird and dark things got.

When Alex got home from his business trip to Germany and saw the level of my physical pain, he understood what I was up against. A week after he returned, I was lying next to him, my pelvic pain throbbing and relentless. I was exhausted but couldn't sleep, and I couldn't stop sobbing. Alex told me that no matter how bad the illness got and no matter what happened, he would always try to help me and never leave me. I was in despair, and his devotion was incredibly comforting.

Alex wanted to know how he could help, so we decided to walk around our neighborhood together each evening. In the privacy of the dark, he would listen quietly as I talked, cried, or vented. He'd encourage me to let out the emotions with him, away from the house, so we could shield the kids from the worst of it. When the pain was at its peak, I would just hang on until he came home, and our walk was the highlight of my day.

One day about four months into the pain, Alex and I ventured out on an errand to Home Depot. As we were standing in the checkout line, my intestines seized up and I made it to the bathroom just in time for a full-on dumping incident. I met Alex at the car and told him what happened.

"We shouldn't leave the house," he said in alarm. But he quickly regrouped and said, "I guess we are just learning how to manage this condition." Then, in his practical way, he added, "Maybe we should get an RV and drive it all over town, so you will always have a bathroom when you need it."

I knew this was an extreme and unnecessary option, but the fact that he was problem-solving and willing to accommodate my needs was so reassuring.

The next week we were on our way to a restaurant when I said, "Maybe I shouldn't go. What if I have another dumping episode?"

"Don't worry. We'll handle it," Alex said. Then, with a mischievous grin, he added, "Let's take my brother's car. We're going to buy it from him soon, and if you have an accident, we can drive down the price!" Alex knew how to use humor to lighten me up, and we had a great night out.

One night a few weeks later, I was in the garage pulling clothes out of the dryer when the tears just started to pour out. Four days earlier Alex had left on a business trip, and since then the pain had been bearing down on me, intense and constant. I felt totally wiped out.

Suddenly, my thirteen-year-old son, Alex, opened the door and looked straight at my wet face and runny nose. He asked me if I were okay. I told him I was tired and hurting a little (a huge understatement), and he reached out and hugged me. As I leaned over his bony shoulders, I shook a little as I repressed a cry, not wanting to lean too heavily on his fragile frame. He asked me if he could help with the laundry, which was an absolute first in that boy's life. When I told him I didn't need help, he picked up the laundry and carried it in.

A few minutes later, he came back and said, "Mom, it is good to let it out. Sometimes, I cry in bed at night when I'm stressed out, and in between classes I try to think of nothing for a few minutes and that helps too." He paused and then said, "I will always be there for you, Mom. I understand you because I'm just like you."

Then, as easily as we had fallen into the depths of connection, we flipped back to normal life. He told me about new postings on YouTube, jokes he'd heard at school, and the feedback he'd received from his teacher on his social studies report. Suddenly aware of the time (my son loves to visit with me at night), I said, "Hey, it's ten o'clock! Get to bed. . . . And thank you so much for helping me."

Sharing the Suffering

When the pain was at its peak during the first few months, I felt completely isolated, as evidenced by this journal entry:

> Sometimes, I feel so alone in my suffering. I want someone to take this pain away from me or suffer with me.

When I shared those feelings with Jackie, she told me that the people who love me are never okay when I am hurting. She said that, even though my loved ones didn't carry the pain physically, they carried it emotionally. Over the next few weeks, a few incidences convinced me that she was right.

One Saturday a few months into the pain, Alex took our son skateboarding and talked to him about my illness. He compared my discomfort to the gas pains my son occasionally experienced, explaining that it was uncomfortable but not terrible and would come and go. He told my son that when I didn't feel well, he could help me out until I felt better.

When they got home, my son bounded through the door and said, "I feel much better, Mom, I thought you were going to die."

In the beginning, when my husband got home from work, he would usually step through the kitchen door, study me, and ask tentatively how I was doing. One day I broke into tears, and told him that the pain had dropped a little but I was terrified it would return. He hugged me and said the pain probably would come back, but he knew I would get better over time. He assured me that we would get through this and I shouldn't worry. I felt better and stopped crying.

Ten minutes later, I peeked around my son's door to call him to dinner. He was sitting at his desk, staring at the blank wall in front of him with his eyebrows knitted and tears on his face. Until then, I hadn't known the effect my suffering was having on his little heart.

As my husband and I were walking one night, I said to him, "You are supportive, but you aren't all emotional about it."

"My getting upset won't help you."

"Do you feel for me?"

The pain welled up in his eyes and transformed his face. He didn't have to say a word.

Knowing that my two guys hurt for me made me feel loved and less alone in my suffering. Four years later, my life coach, Iben told me that when people want others to suffer with them, it is often because they feel completely isolated in their pain and are yearning for some type of emotional connection.

Giving Back

One night on our walk I asked Alex why we talked only about me. He told me that since I was hurting, he didn't want to burden me with anything else, and he felt that, compared with what I was dealing with, his issues seemed tiny. I told him that I may be in pain, but I was still his friend and his wife. Communicating was something I could still do, and in fact, it was one of my core competencies. I told him to not take that away from me and to let me love him back.

From then on, we both had our time to vent on our walks.

When I was in the depths of suffering, the pain would sometimes color my whole life and start to take over my identity. Having people to love and care for helped me to pull out of the pain and to reconnect with other parts of myself.

Setting Boundaries

One night a neighbor I didn't know very well stopped my daughter and me as we were walking in the neighborhood. She talked anxiously and at length about the difficulty of gaining acceptance into good universities, even though both of her girls were attending top schools. As we listened politely, I could feel my buttocks and my entire pelvic floor tighten from the apprehension rising within me. My daughter, Katherine, was just starting high school, and I didn't want this negative conversation to limit her aspirations for the future.

When I told my psychologist, Jackie, about the experience, she advised me to be aware of my reactions to situations and to move away from those that were unpleasant or uncomfortable for me. She said I needed to protect my mental health by minimizing the negative stuff in my life. When negative interactions were unavoidable, she suggested I put up my internal boundaries beforehand to protect my heart. Jackie encouraged me to take care of myself mentally, not only when I was fragile and healing, but always.

The idea that I was responsible for meeting my own mental and emotional needs was new to me. Throughout my life, I'd waited and hoped for others to provide me with love and support, and when those expectations weren't met, I'd felt and held on to resentment. Jackie planted a mental seed that I was in charge of my own happiness.

Throughout my childhood, I was taught that it was my Christian/Catholic duty to put others ahead of myself and to help whenever I was asked. The idea that I should monitor situations and possibly limit how much I gave to other people was completely new. I became willing to consider these ideas only when I was completely depleted and had no other choice.

However, at the time Jackie made that suggestion to me I'd bristled at the idea of putting up an internal boundary. At that point in my healing, I had little appreciation for my internal self and often lived through my contacts with others, so to put up any barrier seemed like spiritual suicide.

Over the years, I would develop more internal resources and learn to set boundaries. Today, creating a boundary feels like wrapping myself in a cocoon that changes in nature from vapor to steel, depending on the situation and the person(s) with whom I am interacting. Within this self-imposed space, my body doesn't need to tighten in protection, and my pelvic area often stays relaxed.

Beyond Achievement

Seeking career challenges used to be my modus operandi. But at the end of 2007, when the semester was over and the debilitating pain was still with me, I quit my teaching job.

On many days, I'd just have to rest. Sometimes, I felt sidelined from life. I had to remind myself that I wasn't unmotivated or lazy; I was resting because my body needed to heal. When I felt good, I had to be careful not to overdo trying to make up for lost time.

Alex advised me, "Set your goals at fifty percent. Then, accept that on some days your productivity will be one hundred percent and on some days it will be zero."

At the beginning of my career as a physical therapist, I'd developed disc problems and pain in my neck. I worried—literally, for two decades—

that these injuries would limit my ability to work with patients, especially because I needed to stay current with my treatment skills in order to teach. But the issue went deeper than simply being worried about how I would make a living. Achieving was my identity. The admiration of patients and students was important to my ego and crucial to my sense of feeling loved. But when the pelvic pain made working impossible, I started to appreciate who I was beyond the jobs I performed and the roles I filled. I'd chosen my career as an expression of my inner person. Yet, it was only when I stopped working that I got to know myself again.

Enjoying Each Day

One day, with the painful road stretched out in front of me like an interminable desert, I just sat there, despairing in the dust. But then, a distinct memory of my mother seeped into my mind, giving me perspective and encouragement to keep plodding along.

It was our last family gathering before my mother died. At that point in her illness, she was almost completely paralyzed, fatigued, and frail but still very much in charge. She directed us (the members of the family gathered there) to move her onto the screened-in porch and to spread out all her jewelry on the table next to her. She instructed each of her children and grandchildren to pick out a piece of jewelry. Then, as she lay motionless on her chaise lounge watching, we slowly took turns, until there was a little pile in front of each of us and the table was empty.

When we carried her back into the house under the glow of the setting sun, she smiled and said, "Now, *that* was a great day!"

Six months into my pelvic pain, I started to adopt my mother's perspective—as expressed in this journal entry:

> Before the pain, I remember being preoccupied with little things, like who won an award at work, how much playing time Katherine got on the basketball team, what I should buy next, a few extra pounds I'd gained. My priorities have changed now that I have limited energy. I have cut out a lot of the unnecessary pursuits in my life, but I am keeping the good stuff. Now, the best and beautiful parts of my life get more attention.

In the pain I'm learning to appreciate the small things in life. I never would have allowed myself time to take a yoga class or to sit in the whirlpool in the daytime. I am now enjoying the little moments alone and with my family. I have stopped running for approval and worrying about achieving, and have just been here to receive love. I'm noticing the blooming plants, and I am blooming where I've been planted. In fact, my life is so much better—if you discount the pain part!

Being of Service

As I was lying in bed reading during my sixth month of pain, I came across the following quote by Eckhart Tolle:

"The acknowledgment of abundance that is all around you awakens the dormant abundance within. Then let it flow out. When you smile at a stranger, there is already a minute outflow of energy. You become a giver. Ask yourself often: 'What can I give here; how can I be of service to this person, this situation?'"

Those words sparked a clear memory of my mother from nine years before. When my parents could still travel, they would leave the cold Chicago winter and spend February at the local beach near my home in Southern California. As we were walking past the shops on Main Street and heading toward the beach on a sunny afternoon during one of my parents' visits, every time we'd pass someone, my mother would look the person in the eye, smile, and say a cheerful "Hello!"

After the third time, I had to set her straight. "Mom, people just don't do that here."

Her voice was kind as she said, "I don't have much to give, but if I can brighten just one person's day with a greeting and a smile, then I need to do it."

A few years later, my mother was too weak to cook for herself, and fellow church members drove thirty minutes to her home in the country three times a week to drop off a meal and to visit. Every day, old and new neighbors and friends would make their way to my mother's home. When I visited her, I would always thank these well-wishers for making this effort on my mother's behalf. They would always tell me they received so much more than they gave in my mother's home.

After my mother died, one of her best friends told me, "I would go to see your mother thinking it was for her. But I was the one who would go home completely filled up and flying high."

On one of the last nights I spent with my mother, I performed the nightly duties: brushing her teeth, putting on her pajamas, and lifting her into bed. As I repositioned her body up in the bed, I miscalculated how much force it would take to move her frail frame and gasped as her head bumped the headboard with a thud. She burst out laughing!

"Mom, how can you be so patient with all of us idiots?"

"I learned a lot from my mother when she had ALS, and I am hoping that is your experience, too."

Then, it hit me. As she was lying there motionless, my mother was still looking for ways to be of service.

In the beginning of my illness when I worried that pain would limit my ability to give to others, I would think about my mom giving in her most powerful way from that hospital bed. She taught me that I could still be useful even if I had chronic pain, and I could still connect with people even when I was suffering.

Making a Difference

On another night about nine months into the pelvic pain, I read the following quote by Eckhart Tolle:

"The great arises out of small things that are honored and cared for. Everybody's life really consists of small things. Greatness is a mental abstraction and a favorite fantasy of the ego. The paradox is that the foundation for greatness is in honoring the small things of the present moment instead of pursuing the idea of greatness. The present moment is always small in the sense that it is always simple, but concealed within it lies the greatest power."

I just had to smile. When I was growing up, I often told my mother that I wanted to achieve something great and make a big difference in the world.

In response, she would always say, "It is in the little things that you make a difference."

One month after I read the Eckhart Tolle quote about greatness, my daughter, Katherine, wrote the following poem for me as a Mother's Day gift.

Ode to the Mother

For you, America has suggested diamonds, cell phones, and clothing
So constant and blunt, these items have brought me to loathing.
Sure these gifts are convenient and fun
But this day's purpose has been undone.
Therefore, for you on this Mother's Day
I have devised a more thoughtful way.

What is it exactly, that makes you so great?
So important, in fact, that you have your own date?
You support your family with love and care
You're always kind and always there.
Each night you prepare a tasty meal
And with every crude joke, you are able to deal.

In the morning, you're consistently cool
You make their lunches and drive them to school
The trip is dull and it is early in the morning,
But you always send their tired spirits soaring.
They may sit in the car, quiet and stern
But you chatter cheerfully around every turn.
Mom, although at times you may be lame,
Life without you would not be the same.

While they're gone in the middle of the day
You attend your appointments as you may.
Sick, hurting, and with lack of rest
You always strive to be your best.
Thanks, Mom, for playing in pain despite the cost
For without you, the game of life would soon be lost.

In the afternoon, when school is out
They call for a ride, without a doubt.
You're always ready; you're rarely late.
You arrive with love and never hate.
You ask about the events of their day

And take in every word they say.
Mom, we appreciate all you do
For in this family, you are the glue.
Connecting Father, Son, and Daughter together,
You ensure we'll stay close forever.

Katherine didn't express these sentiments in everyday life, so I was surprised to see she had that level of awareness and appreciation.

When I shared the poem with Mika Bursch, my first massage therapist at the Healing Sanctuary, he said, "She was helped. There is no way she could know all that." Then he asked, "Who wants you to know you are doing a good job?"

"That would be my mom," I replied. "She always told me I was a good mother."

On my way out, Mika gave me one of his favorite books to borrow: *Simple Truths: Clear and Gentle Guidance on the Big Issues in Life,* by Kent Nerburn.

When I read the book the next week, I found a quote that seemed to have been written especially for me:

"When we come to the end of our journey and the issues that so concerned us recede from us like the day before the coming night, it will be these small touches—the child we have helped, the garden we have planted, the meal we have prepared when we were too weary to do so—that will become our legacy to the universe."

I knew that I could still do the little things even when I was in pain, and now I saw these small acts of kindness as valuable. It was calming to know that even when I was suffering, it was still possible to make a positive difference in the lives of those I loved and in the world.

At the end of my first year of pain, I came across a quote by the authors of *A Headache in the Pelvis* that seemed to summarize how my life and perspective had shifted:

"Learning to live with this pain is about finding what is important in life, less about ego, career, money, status. More about enjoying each day and the quality of your relationships."

3

Climbing Out
of the Pit of Pain

During the first two years of my illness, getting out of physical pain dominated my life. During that time, I tapped into the skills I had gathered from being a physical therapist and a university instructor and tried a plethora of treatments from Western and Eastern medicine.

Years later, I would come to appreciate that this physical breakdown also reflected the state of my overall person and that working through the pain was healing more than my body. In the beginning, however, I did not have this awareness, and my body was hurting so much it demanded my full attention.

In this chapter, I describe my medical condition and the steps I took to try to decrease my pain and cure my condition. Some of these interventions addressed the chronic pain in general, and some specifically targeted the dysfunction of the bladder and pelvic-floor muscles that plagued me. If you are currently in a pit of pain, I hope this chapter gives you ideas and methods that you can use to feel better.

Multi-Faceted Pain

Western medicine excels at analyzing the structure and function of the different systems of the body and parceling out treatment to specialists for each area. For this reason, conditions that affect many systems of the body or have a psychological component, like interstitial cystitis and fibromyalgia, are less understood. In this section, written early in my illness, I describe my signs and symptoms and consider the factors that may have been contributing to my painful illness.

The Bladder

My main symptom was pain in my lower abdomen right above the pubic bone. It felt like I had an extremely full bladder and someone was sitting on my stomach. At the peak of my pain, it was severe, about eight on a scale of one to ten. But after the first few months, the pain settled into the moderate category, ranging from a level four to a level six. At a level four, the pain would interfere with my ability to perform tasks, such as working, exercising, and completing household chores. At a level six, the pain was intense enough that I found it difficult to concentrate. The percentage of the day that I was in pain changed from day to day, but in the first six months of my illness, I was often in pain more than seventy percent of the day.

One day while I was sitting in the waiting room of my physical therapist, Julie, I started talking with another patient, who happened to be a physician. Her pelvic pain originated from an irritation of the pudendal nerve, which is the pelvic nerve that transmits sensation of the external genital areas and controls the sphincters of the bladder and rectum. Because the pudendal nerve supplies so many structures, this woman knew how it felt to have pain at the nerve, muscle, and bladder areas. When I told her that some of my pain was located in the bladder, compassion washed over her face. She told me that of all the pain she had suffered, nothing rivaled bladder pain and it was impossible to ignore at even low levels. She also said that, unlike any other pain, her bladder pain came with a sense that something was not right at a basic level and instigated a primal kind of panic.

That was my experience, too. Even when the bladder pain was mild, it grated on my nerves and ratcheted up my fear and anxiety. Julie explained to me that the bladder has more pain-transmitting nerve fibers than any other organ in the body. Usually, these neurons are silent, but when they wake up, watch out!

Dr. Chalfin performed several tests to determine why my bladder hurt. Urine cultures consistently showed no sign of infection, and my initial ultrasound depicted no structural abnormalities. Only my cystoscopy showed some abnormality—that the interior of the bladder was inflamed.

Pelvic-Floor Muscle Dysfunction

When my internal pelvic muscles would spasm, I'd feel a pulling or tightening sensation anywhere from my pubic bone back to the coccyx (tail bone). Sometimes, I'd feel an intense shooting pain in the vagina, or like a golf ball were stuck in my rectum, or as if my rear end were stuck in a vice. When the external pelvic muscles would spasm, my buttocks and all the muscles around my hip joints would feel achy and tender to the touch. But pain is relative, and although these muscle spasms were uncomfortable, nothing rivaled the bladder pain. I would tell my husband I could endure almost any type of pain except that.

During my pelvic exams at the very beginning of my illness, the doctors and therapists noted my pelvic-floor muscles felt tight and the presence of a deep knot that was as big and hard as a marble. On several occasions, my physical therapist, Julie, put pressure on these internal muscles and reproduced the pain in my bladder. So it was possible that those deep muscle spasms were also contributing to the discomfort in my bladder area.

Musculoskeletal Contributions

Julie told me that many of her pelvic-pain patients stood with their pelvis tipped forward (hip flexion, anterior pelvic tilt, lumbar lordosis). I have always had this posture, and the muscles and nerves in the back of my legs have always been really tight.

Whenever the pelvic pain flared up, the muscles in my body that were often tight became even more taut and tender. For me, the muscles most affected were the superficial and deep gluteals (buttocks), the hamstrings (rear thigh), and the calf (lower-back leg).

When Julie felt my abdomen and upper legs, she noted that the connective tissue (fascia) was often inflexible or thickened. Fascia is the collagenous (elastic) tissue that surrounds all internal structures in the human body, from whole organs to tiny capillaries. Fascial tissue provides support for these structures, separates them, and decreases the friction between them, which is necessary for movement. I have several scars on my abdomen from a hernia surgery and two Caesarean sections, which may have contributed to the fascial restrictions in my pelvic area.

The Nervous System

The connection between my nervous system and my pelvic pain has always been clear to me and my caregivers. When my bladder pain first began, I felt a tingling down my spine, a pulsating energy in my body, and a rhythmic pounding in my ears. When my bladder pain hit high levels or continued for more than a week, my whole nervous system felt like it was buzzing, as if it were ramped up and in overdrive.

After a few months, I started to suspect that the sacral segments of my spinal cord may be overactive, because the bladder and all the muscles with increased tone have neural connections there. I wondered if these neural connections through the spinal cord created a feedback loop between my bladder, nervous system, and the muscles. If so, maybe that is why I had to treat all three before my pain levels dropped. In addition, these spinal-cord segments can be activated from the brain itself. That might be the anatomical explanation for why spinning thoughts and turbulent emotions could ramp up my pain and why I needed to also work at the mental and emotional level to attain long-lasting relief.

Of course, many other parts of the nervous system are also involved in pain transmission. With prolonged pain, these neural-pain pathways can become more prominent and easily excited.

Psychological Factors

Since the whole nervous system is wired together, many connections can influence whether or not the pain pathways are activated. When I was under stress, my pain often increased, and when I was really calm, I could sometimes get the pain levels to drop.

At the very start of my condition, I wondered whether my nervous system had been in overdrive way before the pain began and whether that was another factor that set me up for the condition. Several of my caregivers told me that patients with pelvic pain often have intense, highly productive, "type A" temperaments. That certainly fit my case. Don't get me wrong: Pain should never be explained away based on someone's personality. Many active, intense people never experience pelvic pain. The relationship between my temperament and my pain was complicated, and over time I would understand how they were linked.

Labeling the Symptoms

I was given two diagnoses: (1) interstitial cystitis (IC) and (2) pelvic-floor myopathy (muscular condition or disease) or myalgia (muscular pain). I would find out later that many different labels could be applied to my symptoms, and some researchers and clinicians only use the term IC when cystoscopy reveals ulcerations of the interior bladder walls (Hunner's ulcers). My case could also be labeled as painful bladder syndrome (PBS) or bladder pain syndrome (BPS) or those terms combined with IC (PBS/ IC; BPS/IC). I could also be given the diagnosis of chronic pelvic pain syndrome (CPPS), which is a term originally adopted by researchers of chronic prostatitis, possibly the male equivalent of IC.

Knowing the diagnostic labels for my condition wasn't as helpful as it might have been for illnesses having a well-defined pathology and researched treatments. With my condition, the type and severity of symptoms varies greatly between people with the same diagnoses and even in each individual over time. Even though diagnostic categories are important for medical research and for communication within the medical profession, it was my individual symptoms, rather than my specific diagnosis, that provided the most information about my condition and how to treat it.

An Uncertain Condition

During my first visit to the UC Irvine clinic, Dr. Noblett, the chief urogynecologist, told me that as a resident she'd felt she had a good understanding of IC, but after eight years of working with women with the condition, she now thought it was a complex enigma. She told me that patients with IC often experience different combinations of symptoms, that different pathologies may be underlying the same diagnosis, and that outcomes are difficult to predict.

I had read similar opinions from other medical experts while researching the condition on the Internet. My main symptoms were bladder pain and pelvic-floor tension and pain, but some other patients with a diagnosis of IC experienced frequent urination and bladder sensitivity when they ate certain foods. On cystoscopy, my bladder showed inflammation, but other patients have pinpoint bleeding (glomerulations) or patches of broken skin (Hunner's ulcers), reflecting an actual breakdown of the inner bladder lining. These signs and symptoms could reflect either a more advanced form of the same disease or possibly a whole different disease process. It is possible that many different conditions result in bladder pain and pelvic-floor muscle dysfunction.

Dr. Lane, the other urogynecologist at the clinic, told me that when the medical community doesn't know much about a disease, they often blame it on emotions, and in the past, many doctors had considered IC to be just a sign of emotional hysteria. She said IC is a true pathological condition, but the exact cause and a cure are not yet known.

I blurted out, "Just what you don't want: a painful condition that the medical community doesn't know a lot about!"

Dr. Lane reassured me that more had been learned about IC in the past three years than had been found in the past three decades and that more options would become available in the future.

I thought, *Who cares about the future? I am really hurting now!*

Gathering Theories

I decided to use a multi-dimensional approach and to address many of the possible reasons for my condition all at once. Each of my caregivers gave me possible reasons for why I was in pain—essentially, their individual theories. At first, this was really confusing and I wondered whether they were all just guessing. But really, that is what a theory is: an educated guess. I was subjected to so many different viewpoints because each caregiver looked at my condition through a unique lens, one shaped by their professional training and experience.

Just like my caregivers, I, too, had a biased view of my condition. Probably because of my professional background and what I was experiencing in my own body, I initially found it easiest to accept the pelvic-pain theories that related to a dysfunction of the pelvic-floor muscles and an intensified activation of pain pathways in the nervous system.

Instead of growing frustrated with the barrage of theories about my condition, I decided to tap into these various perspectives in order to figure out how to heal. I found that theories of pelvic pain have various levels of evidence to support them. Some theories are backed up by controlled studies in the research lab, although this is rare. Some theories are recommended from the clinical experiences of physicians and therapists. Others are suggested from positive experiences of patients.

Physical Treatments

When I recount my story to other people, almost everyone asks me what one thing "cured" my condition. Sometimes, they look disappointed when I tell them that, in my case, getting better required a combination of methods from Western medicine, Eastern medicine, and alternative treatments that addressed all aspects of my person—body, mind, and spirit. Their disappointment seems to grow even deeper when I tell them there was no quick fix or cure and the healing happened gradually over time at all levels of my being.

For me, healing chronic pelvic pain was not a simple task. My condition involved many factors, all of which had to be addressed using many different types of treatment before I felt better. Finding the right combination of treatments was often discouraging and frustrating, but with persistence, I found a multi-treatment approach that worked for me.

One indication of how much pain someone is enduring is the extent to which they will go to try to get rid of it. I was in a world of pain. So brace yourself for the long list of measures I took to heal my body.

Diet, Herbs, Supplements

One of the first things the urologist suggested to manage my condition was to adopt the "IC diet," which eliminates foods and drinks that commonly cause irritation of the bladder walls—such as coffee, spicy foods, and citrus juices. I also tried PreRelief®, an over-the-counter medication taken before meals to neutralize acidic foods. Later, my acupuncturist prescribed a combination of Chinese herbs for my condition, which I took in a capsule form called CystiQuell™.

Some researchers postulate that bladder and pelvic pain such as mine (BPS/IC) may result from a general condition that causes inflammation in different parts of the body. They theorize that the same process may underlie many different diseases, including fibromyalgia and irritable bowel syndrome (IBS). Many Eastern and alternative healing approaches suggest changing the diet as a way to decrease inflammation, and this practice is currently gaining interest in Western Medicine, too.

My acupuncturist, Pam, was the first to encourage me to change my diet. She instructed me to add Omega-3 fish oil and Juice Plus+® supplements to my diet in an effort to both increase my nutrition and decrease overall inflammation in my body. Then, she encouraged me to consult a nutritionist and to read the book *The Inflammation-Free Diet Plan,* by Monica Reinagel. Both of these sources emphasized that different foods have varying effects on inflammation throughout the body. I tried changing my diet to include more foods that had low inflammatory ratings—such as fish, vegetables and nuts—and fewer foods with high inflammatory ratings— such as breads and sweets. To keep myself honest, I made a chart listing the foods I commonly ate, their inflammatory rating, and the portion size recommended by the Mayo clinic website and posted it on my refrigerator.

For me, altering my diet was one of the more difficult parts of managing my condition. Even though the information I needed to choose healthy foods was right there on my refrigerator, I often ignored it. I kept eating foods that were highly inflammatory (especially sugar), and not only did I continue to experience bladder pain and other symptoms, but I also gained an extra twenty pounds over the years.

Five years into my illness, I finally got serious about changing my diet. One week, my bladder was irritated for a few days, and I suspected that the flare-up was related to overall body inflammation. In the past when my bladder hurt, my nervous system was ramped up, my pelvic floor was tight, and I was often working through an emotional issue. This time, none of those issues were present. Instead, I felt a heavy discomfort around my stomach, and my body felt bloated.

My physical therapist at the time, Nicole, had just returned from the annual meeting of the International Pelvic Pain Society. She told me two physicians at the conference had made presentations emphasizing the need for patients with chronic pelvic pain to adopt a strict anti-inflammatory diet.

I went to see my life coach, Iben, who had joined my healing team two and a half years into my pain. She, herself, consumed only non-processed, organic, vegetarian foods that were incredibly tasty, and she had been eating that way for over twenty years. Iben gave me many practical suggestions for adopting a healthy eating lifestyle. She advised me to throw out all the sweets in my house that I would be tempted to eat. But, she told me, I would need to transition off the sugar gradually, and suggested that I keep fresh or dried fruit and nuts readily available to satisfy cravings. She told me to set aside time to shop and prepare the food for the week, so healthy options were always available. I changed my diet to include more fruits, vegetables, nuts, and seeds and to cut out refined sugar, red meat, and processed foods. I went online and found recipes that fit my new diet restrictions and bought a blender to make fruit/vegetable drinks.

Iben encouraged me to be easy on myself and not expect to change my diet overnight. She said it is common for people who are trying to adopt healthy eating habits to feel guilty when they don't consume healthy foods or like they're being punished when they refrain from eating foods they crave. She also encouraged me to be aware of the link between my emotions and my eating. She said people often use food to reward themselves or to "fill the hole" when they feel emotionally depleted. That was my common pattern for consuming sweets. Iben explained that as infants, mother's milk (or formula) is the first form of comfort and nourishment and a pacifier is often used to soothe a baby. From this early conditioning, it follows that we often fill our mouth, especially with sweets, to comfort ourselves.

For as long as I can remember, I have always craved sugar, and my addiction to candy is well-known to my family and friends. My mother told me that when I was three years old, she found me on the counter with my head in the cabinets, eating table sugar right from the bowl! Iben told me that in our culture (American), sugar is viewed as something of value and is often used to reward or bribe. One of my clearest memories, from when I was about three, is of my mother promising to buy me candy if I were perfectly good during Sunday mass. Iben encouraged me to become more aware of when I craved sugar and to ask myself if I were using it to numb, stimulate, or substitute.

Just about that time, a friend who is a psychiatrist told me that sugar was a true addiction, and on a functional MRI, sugar lights up the same areas of the brain as do hard-core drugs, like cocaine.

Through all these experiences, I began to see the connections between my diet, my emotions, overall body inflammation, and pelvic pain.

Oral Medications

At the beginning of my illness when the pain levels were at their peak, my internist and family physician, Dr. Ryan, prescribed Cymbalta. This medication is a selective serotonin reuptake inhibitor (SSRI) and a norepinepherine reuptake inhibitor that increases the amount of neurotransmitters between nerve cells. Cymbalta has been shown to decrease nerve pain, chronic musculoskeletal pain, depression, and anxiety. I took Cymbalta for two years, was off it for two years, and then, after my pain ramped up in the spring of 2011, I took it again for one more year. For me, this medication definitely decreased my neurological ramp-up and discomfort when the pain was at high levels or present for a few weeks. The medication did not completely take away the pain; it just calmed down my system so I could deal with it better.

Some experts believe that the blood-thinning (anticoagulant) medication heparin may restore the inner surface of the bladder and protect the bladder wall from substances in urine that could irritate it. In my second month of pain, my urologist, Dr. Chalfin, prescribed an oral derivative of heparin called Elmiron (pentosan polysulfate sodium). It can take up to six months for this medication to be effective, so I took it for that long. When my pain levels had not changed after six months of being treated with Elmiron, I stopped taking it.

Instillations

Initially, Dr. Chalfin used a catheter to insert (instill) DMSO (dimethyl sulfoxide) directly into my bladder. This medication is actually a solvent that made its way into medical use around 1963, when it was found that it could penetrate the skin and carry other components with it into a biologic system. In 1978, a study at the Cleveland Clinic found that DMSO offered significant relief to the majority of the study's 213 patients with genito-urinary disorders. In my case, there was no change in my pain levels after two months of weekly DMSO instillations.

When I went to the clinic at UC Irvine, Dr. Noblett discontinued my use of heparin in the oral form (Elmiron) and directly instilled heparin along with an anti-inflammatory and anesthetic into my bladder.

Many different combinations of medications can be instilled into the bladder, but for me the cocktail was 10,000 units of heparin; 250 milligrams of Solu-Medrol® (methylprednisolone); 2 milliliters of 4 percent lidocaine; and 50 milliliters of sterile water. Each ingredient has a different aim: heparin restores the bladder lining. Solu-Medrol is a steroid that decreases inflammation. Lidocaine is an anesthetic that makes it more comfortable to hold the medication inside the bladder for an hour. Water just gives the cocktail substance.

I endured these instillations every week for two months and then periodically when the pain flared up, for a total of about twenty instillations over the years. At the time, the instillations seemed to decrease my bladder pain slightly for up to a few days. (Later, I would wonder whether it was the lidocaine and/or the steroid, and not the heparin, in the instillation that provided the minor and temporary pain relief.)

Physical Therapy

I found out early on in this journey that it is important to work with a physical therapist who has adequate training and experience in the area of pelvic pain. This type of therapy is not included in the standard curriculum to become a physical therapist, and to learn these advanced skills, therapists often take at least three levels of continuing education courses. Therapists who are designated as a Women's Health Clinical Specialist (WCS) have passed a national exam and have either completed a clinical residency program or had more than 2,000 direct patient-care hours in this specialty area. In addition to this training, it is optimal if the physical therapist has experience working with patients with pelvic pain because treating these conditions requires different skills than treating other conditions in the pelvic area.

My first physical therapist had the WCS title, but she didn't have experience doing internal manual work for the pelvic-floor region or knowledge about pelvic pain. Fortunately, my second physical therapist, Julie, has worked with patients in pelvic pain for almost twenty years. During the more than five years of pelvic pain, I participated in three courses of physical therapy treatment with Julie. The first course began four months into the pain and lasted eighteen months. The second course began two years into the pain and lasted six months. The third course began three and a half years into the pain and lasted over two years.

The fact that I had physical therapy for so much time isn't a sign that the treatments weren't effective. My work with Julie (and later with Nicole) consistently relaxed my pelvic-floor muscles, re-established flexibility in my body, and decreased my pain. However, because my condition had many contributing factors, I had to work at many different levels to consistently stay in a pain-free zone. My physical therapists were a crucial part of this overall healing effort, addressing my physical condition while I uncovered the mental/emotional contributors to the ramp-up of my nervous system and my pain.

On the psychological level, this healing process was like peeling off layers of an onion and progressively healing through them. This same process of working through the layers was mirrored in my body, with deeper and different physical issues surfacing and being addressed over time.

Working at physical and psychological levels simultaneously was crucial for my healing.

As part of my treatment, Julie and later Nicole worked to mobilize tight muscles and fascia throughout my abdomen, back, and upper legs. Each also used her fingers to internally stretch the muscles and fascia of the pelvic floor, accessing these areas through the vagina or rectum. It was similar to having a gynecological exam for close to an hour. As I'm sure any woman would agree, you have to be in real pain to agree to this type of therapy! Obviously, it is also important to have a therapist who is knowledgeable, skilled, trustworthy, and compassionate, and Julie and Nicole are all of those.

During these treatments, my therapists often detected taut bands or nodules in my muscles, called trigger points, that were very tender. When Julie or Nicole applied gentle pressure to a trigger point for a few minutes, the tension in the area often normalized and the pain decreased.

In addition to manual work, Julie provided me with transcutaneous electrical nerve stimulation (TENS). This machine produces a tingling sensation that competes with pain transmission up the spinal cord, so it helps mask the pain. Electrodes are placed either over the bladder, down the spine, or on the lower back and leg in the sacral nerve-root distribution.

Occasionally, Julie performed either micro-current electrical stimulation or cold laser treatments. For each modality, an applicator is moved over the lower abdomen in an attempt to decrease inflammation and accelerate healing of the bladder.

In addition, my therapists evaluated the posture, movement patterns, flexibility, and strength throughout my body and treated those areas that were contributing to my pelvic pain. They also gave me a home program and helped me to progressively increase my activity and exercise while monitoring the effect of this activity on my pelvic pain.

Home Treatments

Diligently attending my physical therapy appointments wasn't enough. I also needed to work on my own every day to maintain the gains made during therapy. Julie instructed me on how to internally stretch the muscles of my pelvic floor and how to apply pressure on trigger points using my fingers or a tool called a "crystal wand." She also showed me how to perform self-massage of muscles throughout my body, especially those at my lower back, hips, and upper legs that directly contributed to my pelvic-floor muscle tightness. For this purpose, I learned to use my hands and other tools, such as foam rollers, small balls, or a hand-held, heated, vibrating massager.

In order to relax the pelvic muscles, I would often sit in a warm or hot whirlpool. I squatted on the seat of the whirlpool with my feet on the seat and moved my body so the water jets would pulsate on my lower spine (lumbar spine and sacrum), butt muscles (gluteals), or the back of my hip joints where the gluteal muscles attach.

Julie also encouraged me to breathe primarily with my diaphragm and to become more aware of the rising and falling of the lower abdomen that occurs with this type of breathing. Diaphragmatic breathing is deeper and slower than chest breathing, and this helps calm the nervous system. In addition, as the diaphragm descends, the pelvic-floor muscles often automatically relax and lengthen.

Massage Therapy

To address areas of my body that were difficult to reach and persistently tight, I worked with a massage therapist, Chris. She performed deep-tissue massage to decrease muscular tension and painful trigger points throughout the body, especially in the muscles that attach to the pelvis.

Suppositories

When my pelvic-floor muscles were not releasing their grip during my first course of physical therapy, Dr. Noblett prescribed a suppository form of the muscle relaxant Baclofen®, which a compounding pharmacy made to her specifications. When inserted into the vagina or rectum, this medication decreases nerve activation and secondarily relaxes muscles.

Three years into the pain when Baclofen was not effective, I also tried a suppository form of the medication Valium® for a few months to aid muscle relaxation. Many of Dr. Noblett's patients benefit from these medications, but they seemed not to decrease the tension in my pelvic-floor muscles.

Pelvic-Floor Trigger-Point Injections

When my pelvic-floor muscles were still not letting go during my first course of physical therapy, Dr. Noblett injected them with a combination of the topical anesthetics Marcaine® (bupivacaine) and lidocaine. To do this, she put a long needle up through my vagina and inserted it into the muscles of the pelvic floor or the area around the pudendal nerve. This was immediately followed by physical therapy in an attempt to break the cycle of pain and spasm. I endured this uncomfortable procedure only because I was in major pain! But these shots were not as bad as they sound. My physicians were skilled, and the deep areas of the pelvic floor have much less sensation than the more superficial areas of the perineum.

Many of these treatments sound painful and invasive, and sometimes they are. But the skill and compassion of my caregivers made them much easier to endure.

Alternative Treatments

Before this illness, I would roll my eyes at treatments that were not based in Western medicine. I remember being in a seminar many years ago, when I was teaching, in which the presenters described some alternative treatments, such as the Feldenkrais and Trager approaches. I, along with my colleagues, challenged the lecturers to provide evidence of treatment efficacy, and we discounted their ideas as nonsense. But the chronic and intense pelvic pain motivated me to be more open-minded and to try different healing options.

Each of my Western medicine doctors encouraged me to combine their efforts with alternative treatments. Dr. Ryan told me that some patients will take medication but are not open to alternative medicine, while others will only go the alternative route and won't consider taking medication. She said the reason I had such a good outcome was because I was willing to try options from Western, Eastern, and alternative medicines. To my surprise, when I tried treatments outside of Western medicine, I had interesting and positive healing experiences.

Yoga

With my urologist, Dr. Chalfin's, encouragement, I attended a yoga class at my gym. I didn't have high expectations because I had tried the class a few months before my pain began and hadn't liked it. I thought the pace was too slow, and I got frustrated at how inflexible I was compared with everyone else around me.

The second time I tried the yoga class, I was at a point in my illness when the pain screamed for my attention most of the day. So I was shocked when I was pain-free throughout the class. This happened consistently, so during the first eighteen months of pain, I attended a yoga class taught by Stella Tryon three times a week.

Then, after Stella stopped teaching at the gym and was replaced with another instructor, I realized not all classes and instructors are alike and how lucky I had been. Stella's class had the right emphasis and pacing to quiet my pain.

I was also surprised to find out that there are different types of yoga. I chose to learn and practice hatha yoga, in which you move into and hold different body postures. But even hatha yoga classes can be vastly different, depending on the style and emphasis of the instructor. Some classes have a yang emphasis (active, masculine energy) and include a flow of poses that work on flexibility, strength, and balance. Others have a yin emphasis (quiet, feminine energy) and include long-held poses that increase flexibility, especially in the spine, hips, and pelvic area. Some classes combine both yang and yin types of energy/activity.

My acupuncturist, Pam, told me that yoga was meant to restore energy (chi, ch'i, or qì) to the body and should not be stressful or competitive. She encouraged me to listen to my body, and when I needed a rest, to just stop and imagine the sequence.

Child's pose is always a good resting posture for me because it tends to relax and stretch my pelvic-floor muscles. Yin yoga is also very beneficial for me because it is slower paced and includes long-held poses that stretch my tight areas.

In yoga, the movements of the body are synchronized with one's breathing. This was crucial to my relaxation and pain relief.

For me, the most important features of a good yoga class are a peaceful atmosphere, a pace that doesn't flare me up, and good breathing cues. Over time, yoga became a moving meditation, a way to quiet my mind by focusing on my body sensations and my breath.

Reiki

When I was resting in corpse pose (savassana) at the end of yoga class, Stella would place her scented hands near my head. Whenever she did this type of aromatherapy, I felt some kind of heat or energy between her hands and my head. One day after class, I asked Stella about other natural healing methods, because I was reading a book about it. She talked to me for forty-five minutes about all types of alternative healing, including Reiki, of which she was a practitioner.

As we headed to our cars, I asked Stella if she would work with me. Being open to alternative treatments and inviting a stranger into my home was totally out of character for me, but I was in pain and desperate. A few days later, there she was—an exotic-looking yogi and Reiki master, dressed in a leotard, her brown hair in pigtails, standing in my living room.

During that first Reiki treatment, I laid face down on a blanket on the floor of my living room, beaten down with pain. When Stella placed her hands near the left side of my head, I felt a vibrating energy moving between her hands and my head, and much to my surprise, I started to sob! Although I didn't feel particularly sad, the tears flooded out like a rainstorm, soaking the blanket beneath me.

Then, Stella pressed her fingers deep into the soles of my feet, and I felt a pulsating beat right in my bladder. I remember wondering if the sensation on the weight-bearing surfaces of the feet was processed in the same segment of the spinal cord as the bladder and if that was how those feelings were related. (Obviously, I wasn't very good at quieting my mind and relaxing.)

Afterward, I reported to Stella what I'd felt during the session. She told me she had placed her hands over my feet but had never touched them.

Another unexpected outcome was that my bladder stopped hurting during the Reiki session and the pain relief lasted into the next day.

Since then, I have had numerous Reiki sessions. My response has never been as extreme as that first session, but I almost always feel warmth and gentle pulsations or tingling in my body, accompanied by an immediate decrease in pain that lasts up to a few days.

The theory behind Reiki treatments is that Universal energy moves through the body of the Reiki practitioner and transfers from his or her hands into the body of another person. This energy is thought to accelerate the natural healing process.

My massage therapist, Chris, is also a Reiki master. She told me that Reiki masters enable others to become clear conduits for this energy by providing "attunements" to open up the internal channels in the body. She said that during this process I would feel her hands placed lightly on specific places on my body. After hearing this explanation, I knew I had definitely strayed outside the boundaries of Western medicine and would find little or no hard evidence to back up these ideas.

Even though I was very skeptical, I couldn't deny that Reiki consistently calmed my nervous system and decreased my pain. So I decided to go through the attunement process because I wanted to be able to treat myself. After going through the procedure, I would rest with my hands over my lower abdomen and focus on sending healing energy to that area on a daily basis.

Over the years, my body responses to Reiki and other energy work would become increasingly obvious and immediate. In addition, after receiving the Reiki attunements, when I would perform manual physical therapy techniques on people, they often reported they felt heat or vibration under my hands.

Meditation

One day in the third month of pain, my friend Sandy dropped off her son at my house. Our boys have been best friends for many years, and Sandy and I always fell into deep conversation whenever we met through them. Sandy's eyes flashed with compassion as she witnessed the pain bearing down on me, and she encouraged me to try meditation. She had been meditating for about a year and had experienced the benefits of this peaceful state of internal awareness. At the time, I instead chose to stay curled up with a heating pad, watching trashy television shows.

Over the years, the encouragement to meditate kept flowing in from other people. Eventually, I began to incorporate meditation into my treatment plan.

I met another pelvic-pain patient who had attended a seminar put on by the authors of *A Headache in the Pelvis*. During the seminar, this patient had practiced paradoxical relaxation using a series of audiotapes, and she let me borrow a few of them. With this type of meditative practice, I would focus on a specific body area, feel the muscle tension, try to let go of the tension, and then stay quiet and focused, accepting whatever happened. In accepting whatever tension remained, I relaxed even further. Sometimes, I would contract the muscles before relaxing them to help my mind cue in to that part of my body.

Then, my acupuncturist, Pam, gave me a CD: *Guided Imagery to Enhance Healing for Women with Pelvic Pain, Interstitial Cystitis or Vulvodynia*, by the Beaumont Women's Initiative for Pelvic Pain and Sexual Heath. I used this CD a few times to help guide the relaxation of my body. Even though the CD was good, I found that I relaxed more when I created the images myself and they were directly related to what I was feeling in my own body.

About eighteen months into my illness, Sandy brought me to her yoga class, which combined meditation with long-held yoga poses that stretched out the hips and pelvic area (yin yoga). We attended the class together every week for about six months. This class emphasized mindfulness meditation, in which you focus awareness on one aspect of your experience, such as body sensations, emotions, or stimulation from the environment. The key is to accept your experience without evaluating or analyzing it and limiting the attention given to the constant stream of thoughts parading through the mind.

Several of my practitioners encouraged me to focus on one thing in order to clear my mind of all other thoughts. When my mind started to wander, I was to return to this focal point. Stella suggested using the flame of a candle as a focal point; Julie recommended using a repeated phrase (mantra). Later, my life coach, Iben, instructed me to sit in a chair and focus on my breathing every morning and every evening, starting with five minutes per sitting and increasing the time as I felt comfortable.

Through all these experiences over the first two and a half years of pain, I gradually stepped into a meditation practice. I found that meditation isn't something to be accomplished or achieved. It is a natural state of being that is available to anyone, requiring only that you quiet the mind and just "be." It takes time to be able to do this. The key is to keep practicing and not get too frustrated with yourself when your mind wanders.

Now, I can quickly quiet my mind and go into a meditative state, which is different than being awake or asleep. It is hard to explain how it feels to rest in this alert, yet quiet, state. But for me, learning how to calm my spinning mind and to rest peacefully has been completely worth the effort, and its benefits are obvious. Meditating calms my mind, my nervous system, and my pain.

Acupuncture

In the sixth month of pain, Dr. Noblett and Julie recommended that I work with Pam, an acupuncturist who specialized in pelvic pain.

Before the pain began, the thought of having needles placed in my body would have sent me running in the opposite direction. At this point, however, I welcomed any opportunity to relieve my discomfort. To my surprise, my first acupuncture treatment was a pleasant experience, and over time, I actually looked forward to my visits.

I hardly noticed the insertion of the tiny needles because Pam always kept me talking. Once the needles were placed, I would rest for about thirty minutes with a relaxed body and quiet mind, and sometimes I fell asleep. Occasionally, I would feel a light tingling in different parts of my body.

Pam kept detailed notes on how I was progressing in all aspects of my healing. She also provided Chinese herbs, supplements, and counseling related to my diet. On each visit, she re-evaluated me and fine-tuned the needle placement. I almost always felt pain-relief during the treatment, and the relief would last from several hours to several days afterward.

The aim of acupuncture is to restore and balance the energy (chi) in the body. This process often takes time, so the treatment is not considered a quick fix. In my case, over the course of about thirty acupuncture treatments, the pain levels gradually decreased until I was pain-free. After that point, I would revisit acupuncture when I had an occasional flare-up to get me back into the pain-free range. During my first bout with pelvic pain, I attended one hundred acupuncture sessions.

Several years later when my pain flared up again, I returned to Pam for more acupuncture because it had been highly effective in decreasing my pain previously. However, during this second flare-up three years into my illness, my nervous system ramped up and my bladder pain increased after each of three acupuncture sessions. Dr. Ryan hypothesized that my threshold of perception had probably dropped because of all the energy work I had done. She was right, and at that point in my healing, subtler forms of energy work, like Reiki, were more effective in decreasing my pain.

Listening to the Body

Over the first two years of pain, I realized my body was giving me information about the cause of my condition and how to treat it. When I became aware of the factors that increased my pain and the treatments that decreased it, the nature of my individual pain condition became clearer.

Using Flare-Ups as Clues

During the first year of pelvic pain when my pain levels were high, my caregivers often asked, "What do you think flared you up?"

I had no response, because I was flared up all the time and it was hard to know what was causing it. At that point, I was just trying different treatments hoping they would lessen the pain.

However, when the pain started to drop and I had some periods of less pain or no pain, the cycles were easier to determine. Each time the pain ramped up, I asked myself, *What changed that may have pushed me into the painful region?* Keeping a list of this information from many different flare-ups and looking for common factors helped me better understand my condition.

Learning from the Treatment Response

In the beginning of my illness, although the pain and dysfunction were obvious, the reason for those problems was unclear. But over the years, my responses to different treatments gave me information about the underlying cause of my condition.

When my bladder was painful, the DMSO instillations and taking heparin orally definitely did not decrease my pain, and having heparin instilled with a catheter had only a minimal effect on my discomfort. In addition, my bladder pain didn't usually fluctuate with what I ate or drank. These experiences provided evidence that a breakdown of the inner lining of the bladder was not the primary cause of my pain.

In contrast, my bladder pain often dropped when my physical therapist released the tension in my pelvic-floor muscles, and on a few occasions she even reproduced my bladder pain by putting pressure on an internal muscle or nerve. These experiences provided evidence that my bladder pain was related more to a musculoskeletal and/or neurological issue rather than to a deteriorating organ. The involvement of my nervous system was further confirmed when calming treatments (such as yoga, meditation, and Reiki) effectively decreased my pain.

Sometimes when I was working through a difficult emotional issue in therapy, my bladder pain would automatically surface or my pelvic-floor muscles would tighten. Then, after I had worked through my deepest stuff, my body would settle down. From these experiences, it became clear that there was a strong emotional component to my pain.

Later, treatments that worked at the mind-body level (Myofascial Release and CranioSacral therapy) were highly effective in relieving my pain. This provided some evidence that my condition was more systemic rather than a dysfunction of one particular body part and that it was also related to the relationship between my mind and body.

Recording and Reporting

As a physical therapist, I loved when patients were able to clearly describe their pain and how it affected their lives. This information helped me develop a plan for their care and evaluate the effectiveness of my interventions. Now, as a patient, I wanted to give my caregivers accurate information so they could make good decisions on my behalf. In this section, I share the strategies I used to understand my condition and communicate with my caregivers.

Charting Pain

After I had been in pain for about six months, my husband made a spreadsheet for me (Appendix 2), and each night I would chart my experience for the day. Little did I know that something so simple would be so important to both me and my caregivers in understanding my condition and how to treat it. Appendix 2 includes two examples of my spreadsheet: one from six months into my illness and another a full year later. These charts provide a concrete representation of how my symptoms improved over the first two years.

My chart included my daily pain level for both the bladder and the pelvic-floor area and my frequency of urination. I recorded the medications I took each day, when I had an instillation, my activities (such as yoga), and my treatments (such as physical therapy and psychotherapy). This data helped me figure out which factors cycled with my pain and so might be important as well as which treatments consistently helped to decrease my pain.

In addition, charting my pain gave me a graphic representation of my progress over time. With my condition, the changes were gradual, and progress tended to wax and wane. So I had difficulty appreciating how I was doing on a day-to-day basis, and honestly, when I was in pain, nothing was clear. But when the changes were viewed month to month or year to year, the general trend of my condition became obvious.

Sometimes, the pain would be so intense or so prolonged that I would lose perspective. So, if I were having a hard time, I'd look at my chart and understand my emotional reactions better. Several times I felt like I was losing control, and when I looked at the data, I reassured myself, *The pain has been high for several days; it's just wearing you down.*

At every visit and often many times a week, a different caregiver would ask, "How have you been doing since our last visit? How is your pain?" Things often fluctuated a lot during the week, and I didn't want to have to remember all that information. So every night I rated my pain and symptoms on my chart. Then, to answer my caregiver's question, I just showed them my chart or summarized the data verbally.

I also brought my spreadsheet to my monthly follow-up visits with my different caregivers. Instead of just a general idea of whether my pain was worse, the same, or better, my caregivers could see my pain in a clear, objective, and graphic form. They all loved it. When Dr. Ryan entered the treatment room, her first words to me were often, "Where's my chart?"

Being a Historian

In my second month of pain, Dr. Ryan, my internist and general practitioner, told me, "I just talked with Dr. Chalfin, and he told me you were a great historian."

"Oh, he probably thought I was so intense. I typed up my whole history," I said.

"Are you kidding? Having all that information saves so much time."

On my first visit with a new doctor or therapist, I would always bring a typed copy of my medical history. (Appendix 2 lists the type of information I included in my medical history.)

Sometimes, the caregiver asked a series of questions, and I used my write-up to make sure I relayed the important information. Other times, the caregiver simply asked me to tell my history, and then I used my notes to highlight the main points in an organized fashion. Many of my doctors liked to review a copy of the medical history I brought as I narrated the main points, and some put it directly into my medical records.

Describing Pain

About six months into the pain, my acupuncturist, Pam, was ready to taper off my visits because my pain levels were low and seemed to be dropping. I thought, *Hmm, why is this not matching my true experience?* Then, I realized I'd been reporting less pain than I was actually feeling because I wanted to show improvement to please my caregivers as well as to convince myself that I was getting better!

My first massage therapist at the Healing Sanctuary, Mika, overheard this conversation between Pam and me, and when Pam left the room, he approached me. He encouraged me to be completely honest about my pain no matter what the levels were so I would get the care I needed in order to get better. I decided to take Mika's advice. To keep myself honest, I began to consistently use the Universal Pain Assessment Tool to quantify my pain. For me, the "activity tolerance scale" of this commonly used measure of pain was the most objective, and therefore, the most helpful. Appendix 2 lists the characteristics I commonly used to accurately describe my pain.

Making an Action Plan

About six months into my illness, I made an action plan and updated it about once a month (see Appendix 2). My action plan had three parts. The first part included daily tasks to manage the condition. I would often forget or get lazy and not follow through on the pain-management strategies, especially when I felt good. Using this checklist kept me on track most of the time.

The second part of the plan listed what I should do when I flared up. This was important, because when the pain would cycle up, I often panicked and this list gave me concrete actions to take when I wasn't thinking clearly.

The third part of the plan gave me new things to try, which helped me to focus on moving forward, especially when I felt like I wasn't getting better.

The benefits of having an action plan were more than just physical. Being proactive had positive mental and emotional benefits, too. The first line of action gave me control, the second gave me peace, and the third gave me hope.

Decreasing Mental Management

I tried to off-load the mental work of managing my physical illness whenever possible. Dealing with chronic pain was tough enough!

Even simple things, like putting all of my appointments on a central calendar and placing my medications/supplements in an organizer with compartments for each day of the week, decreased the mental load considerably. In addition, every time I had a question or concern that I wanted to relay to my caregivers, I put it on a running list, so I didn't have to keep it in my mind until the next appointment.

When I didn't have to remember every detail of my physical condition and medical management, my mind could rest. Identifying with the illness was stressful for my body, and the more I could give my mind a break, the better it was for my physical healing.

Researching My Condition

When I found out that I may have IC, I immediately went online to read a few scientific studies and online postings. Almost all the information I found increased my anxiety and pain. Most of the time, I couldn't even get past the abstract. A line like, "Interstitial cystitis is a chronic, disabling condition," would stick in my head and suck the hope out of me for days.

My journal entry during the second month of my pain depicts how this research destabilized me:

> *Dr. Chalfin tells me this is the worst the pain will get, but I've read that IC can be a progressive disease and the pain can be worse than end-stage cancer. He tells me many women lead normal lives, but I've read that IC can be extremely debilitating, with disability rivaling that of patients on kidney dialysis. Is he telling me the truth? Am I being realistic or catastrophic with my thinking?*

Gathering information had been my modus operandi as a college instructor, but now it just ratcheted up my fear and exacerbated my pain. I found lots of information I could weave into my worst-case scenario. So, early in my illness, I decided to stop researching my condition and to just work closely with my caregivers and monitor the responses of my body.

I also decided that if I researched my condition again, I would use the following guidelines from the book *A Headache in the Pelvis* to figure out whether new information should get my attention:

> *"If the theory about your condition carries some course of action or treatment to help you without unacceptable risks, then it may be an idea that merits your careful consideration. You may wish then to investigate the efficacy of such a course of treatment along with the risks and costs."*

Joining Support Groups

In the first few months of my illness, I joined a few online chat groups that were meant to support women with IC. I quickly found out that having the same diagnosis as other patients didn't necessarily mean that sharing with them would be helpful. When I'd read the online postings of other sufferers, I would add their issues to my own worst-case scenario, and my anxiety would mount. When others in my situation wallowed, vented, or complained, my pain intensified and my future seemed bleak. I just didn't have enough light within myself to keep out of that dark place.

This is not to say that you can't have wonderful relationships with other patients. My physical therapist, Julie, introduced me to a few of her patients who were proactive and positive. Each of these women was generous with advice and encouragement, and finding someone who actually knew what I was feeling was refreshing.

One woman lent me several meditation tapes without ever meeting me. When I thanked her profusely, she said, "We are fighting the same battle. How could I not help out a fellow comrade?" Of all the encouragement I received, hers gave me the most hope because she was walking in my shoes.

Now, I use the same criteria for interacting with other patients as I employ when choosing my friends. I move away from relationships that deplete me and move toward relationships that nurture and uplift me.

Physical Healing

During the first two years of intense pain, there were ups and downs, good days and bad. But over time, the general trend of my condition became clear: I was healing. At the start, the bladder pain was debilitating, intense, and constant. Over two years, the bladder pain became less intense and intermittent, and the duration of my pain-free episodes gradually lengthened. Initially, the muscle spasms were deep within the pelvic floor and the knot inside was hard as a rock, but eventually, the muscle spasms softened and the knot dissipated.

I gradually weaned off physical therapy, psychological counseling, and prescription medication, and I reduced my acupuncture treatments from once a week to just once a month for maintenance. From an anatomical standpoint, my body seemed to be healing from the inside out. From a chronological perspective, my body seemed to be reversing the direction of dysfunction, with the newer and more intense symptoms, like bladder pain, resolving first, and the older and more persistent problems, like postural malalignment, changing more slowly over time.

4

The Other Side of the Treatment Table

I had been a physical therapist for over twenty years when my pain began, and it was very eye-opening to experience the patient-care dynamic from the other side of the treatment table. I was a confident clinician, but as a patient in major pain, I was initially passive and timid.

It took years for me to develop my own power and to function as an equal partner with my caregivers. As a clinician, I thought the patient-care dynamic was important, but it wasn't until I was a patient myself that I really understood how powerful these interactions could be. Sometimes, these exchanges impacted my healing more powerfully than the physical treatments a caregiver provided.

Beyond Embarrassment

In the third month of pain, I emailed a colleague of mine to see if she knew of a good physical therapist who treated the pelvic region.

She wrote back, "I'm so sorry to hear that you are having such discomfort. This might be especially uncomfortable, since it's not pleasant to discuss bodily functions with all these people."

I remember wondering, *Should I be embarrassed? Are other people looking at me differently because I have pain in the pelvic area?*

Then, I remembered teaching at Western University of Health Sciences about six months before my pain began. There was a course in the adjacent classroom called Gynecologic Visceral Manipulation, and as I walked by and saw the overhead of the bladder on the wall, I remember thinking how weird that type of physical therapy was and how I would never treat someone with that problem. Without even knowing it, I had adopted the convoluted views of society about the pelvic region and the natural functions related to this area.

My perspective changed completely when I began suffering from pelvic pain. I was housed in this body, and the pelvic area was simply another part of me. And now it was screaming for my attention! I thought to myself, *You don't need to be embarrassed. You just need compassionate help.*

Crucial Compassion

During my first psychotherapy visit with Jackie, she told me she felt really sorry for me, and I could see the empathy in her eyes. She knew what I was enduring because she herself had suffered with cystitis for a full year.

Yet, my initial response to her empathy had been to reject it. I thought, *Quit feeling bad for me! I'm trying to handle this pain and hold myself together here!* This reaction came not from inner strength but from fear; I was doggedly ignoring the pain and trying in vain to hide from it.

Jackie encouraged me to be honest and realistic about the painful place I was in. She supported me and helped me to build up my inner strength so I could keep walking on this difficult journey.

In the second month of my illness—the pinnacle of pain—I sat on the papered treatment table facing Dr. Ryan. "This pain is worse than the nerve pain I felt when I ruptured the disc in my neck," I said. "It's so bad I sometimes feel like a caged animal."

When I saw tears in Dr. Ryan's eyes, I thought I must be imagining things. But over the years, I saw her tear up a few more times. For me, experiencing compassion and being seen as a whole person was healing in its own right.

Taking Control

After three months of diet changes, medications, and instillations, my pain levels were still through the roof. I remember sitting on my psychologist, Jackie's, couch in pain and in tears.

After studying me for a moment, she said, "You are talking like your condition will never get better. You don't have to resign yourself to a life of pain."

Jackie told me I was in charge of the effort to heal myself and I needed to try all avenues to get better. She said I was responsible for choosing with whom I wanted to work, and if I was working with someone who wasn't helping me, I had to move on and find someone who was helpful. This was true even for my relationship with her, she said; if I felt my sessions with her weren't meeting my needs, she expected me to find another therapist.

Jackie's pep talk was a turning point for me, and I became more proactive in my own healing process. I found Julie and the UC Irvine clinic that specialized in my condition along with other people to help and guide me.

About this time the sentence, "Get into your healing!" jumped out at me from the last paragraph of Catherine M. Simone's book, *Along the Healing Path: Recovering from Interstitial Cystitis*. That one comment from another person who suffered with IC gave me hope that I could get better, put me in charge of the healing effort, and inspired me to keep going.

Dr. Ryan told me that patients who improve have a similar attitude. They see their illness as an issue to work through and get past because they want to go on with the rest of their life. They seek out the care they need, listen to caregivers they trust, and follow through with the plan.

I wondered, *What if I have desire and commitment, and I still don't get better?*

Then I told myself, *You stack the odds of healing in your favor if you continue to do everything you can and don't give up.*

Choosing Teammates

Over time, I learned my preferences in the patient-care dynamic. I wanted to be considered an equal team member, and I wanted the caregiver to value my input, be personal, and listen as well as direct me.

But not every person I worked with dealt with me in this optimal way.

I was never happy when a caregiver took on a formal tone, didn't really listen, or put me in a passive role. It was obvious when the person caring for me didn't have compassion, even if they were outwardly polite. Working with someone with chronic pelvic pain requires exceptional emotional awareness, and not everyone has that gift. I found that a person who has intelligence and skills in the medical arena doesn't necessarily have good interpersonal skills.

In the beginning, when the interaction with a caregiver didn't meet my expectations for emotional support, I would redouble my efforts to connect with him or her on a personal level. If they said something I didn't agree with or that was completely offensive, I just politely smiled and took it in. In some ways I felt at the mercy of my caregivers and thought I needed to be liked in order to get good care.

Over time, I realized that my caregivers were just people, and not all of them would be a good fit for me on a personal level. If I had to put up a protective boundary in any way, I knew the treatment the person provided would be less effective for my healing. I realized that one of the most crucial criteria for a teammate was whether they were healthy for me on an emotional level.

Team Manager

At first I took a subordinate role when working with my caregivers and tried hard to please them. For example, after my first bladder instillation, I told my urologist, Dr. Chalfin, that, even though it was really uncomfortable, I held the medication inside my bladder for a whole hour. He frowned and told me that keeping DMSO inside for more than fifteen minutes could cause bladder irritation. I didn't have the guts to tell him that his nurse had instructed me to keep the medication inside for as long as I could tolerate it.

This need to please my caregivers was challenged early in my illness. When Dr. Chalfin sent me to physical therapy at the UC Irvine clinic, he informed Dr. Noblett and me that he would continue to follow my case. However, when I started therapy, I realized that the clinic also offered interventions and a team approach that fit my needs. I wanted to transfer my care to the doctors there, but my physical therapist, Julie, was uncomfortable with that plan. She worried that physicians in the community would not send people to physical therapy at the UC Irvine clinic if it meant they'd lose their patients. Even though I knew that transferring my care was in my best interests, I didn't do it right away because I was afraid of offending Dr. Chalfin or Julie.

I told Dr. Chalfin about my positive experiences at the clinic, hoping he would get the hint that I wanted to transfer my care. When he didn't react, I resigned myself to staying with him, even though he had stopped taking my insurance. But as he was leaving the treatment room, he turned and said, "If you want to be seen over there, it is fine with me." Only then, with his approval, did I feel free to move on.

This need to please my caregivers continued at the UC Irvine clinic. Months later, during several instillations, my pelvic-floor muscles went into a spasm and pushed out the whole catheter before the medicine could be put in. The catheter then had to be reinserted, which was very painful. This happened three times with different nurses, and each time I laid there enduring in silence.

About nine months into my illness, I finally took control. Before the procedure, I told a new nurse what usually happened and what had worked in the past to prevent the problem. Then, when the procedure went well, I thanked her for listening. After several experiences like this, I started to realize that I had valuable information to share with those working with me.

Gradually, over the first year of pain, I became an active participant in my healing team and put myself in the role of manager. I was able to switch perspective because the pain subsided a bit and I realized I had many treatment options. I felt less like a vulnerable child accepting whatever was given and more like an adult choosing the services I wanted.

When I took control mentally, I was no longer constrained by the perspective of one caregiver. I could be creative, gathering up different ideas and combining them into a treatment plan that fit me. I still listened to my trusted teammates and almost always followed their advice, but I also knew that, ultimately, I was in charge of my healing.

Dealing with Uncertainty

I wanted my doctors to know exactly what to do to stop my pain and to give me a guarantee that I'd get better. But that wasn't possible with my condition.

In response to my questioning, my family doctor, Dr. Ryan, would smile warmly and say, "Sorry, I don't have a crystal ball in here. This condition would be so much easier to handle if you had a guarantee that you would be better, even if you knew it would take years to get there."

This lack of resolution constantly reminded me that the human body is complicated and we are just at the beginning stages of understanding how it works and its potential for healing.

Faced with this uncertainty, my thoughts would swing from negative to positive. Sometimes, I would despair that there was no hard evidence about what the problem was and how to fix it. I remember telling my friend that I would rather have breast cancer than IC, because even though cancer may be life-threatening, the medical community knows more about it and there are more treatment options. When you have cancer, people also understand what you are going through, so you get more support.

I never told Dr. Ryan about this conversation with my friend. So her comments at my next appointment were surprising and reassuring: "IC isn't like some cancers, where the outcome is grim. This condition isn't static, and it can change over time."

Looking at it from that perspective, the fact that no one knew the true outcome was actually hopeful. If the outcome was uncertain, there was a chance it could turn out well.

This point of view was reinforced by two inspirational quotes I read in a newsletter that arrived at our house during that difficult period:

"In the face of uncertainty, there is nothing wrong with hope."

— Bernie Siegel

"Hope sees the invisible, feels the intangible, and achieves the impossible."

— Charles Caleb Colton

Keeping My Power

During the first year of my illness, I met with Jackie, Pam, and Julie at least once a week. Even though they never spoke to one another, on some weeks they would all tell me the same thing but from different perspectives. When I heard the same idea from all three of my caregivers, I knew I should perk up my ears and listen. Jackie, my psychologist, observed that I was now going to different sources and taking in what was right and healing for me.

Words are powerful. They can invoke hope or despair, especially when an authority speaks them and you are in pain.

Here are some of the conflicting messages I received during the first painful year and how those words affected me:

First physical therapist: "I'll do my best to help you feel better, but if you have IC, there is not much I can do for you." . . . *Despair.*

Julie, my second physical therapist: "From my gut, my experience, and your progress, I believe you will be one hundred percent healed." . . . *Hope!*

Dr. Ryan: "You need to look at the glass as half full and not half empty. Sometimes, we can get people to only forty percent, and they have to be thankful it is not worse." . . . *Despair.*

Dr. Ryan: "You will get past this. It's like a rock in your path—more like a huge boulder—but you'll find a way around it." . . . *Hope!*

Nurse: "We will never be able to get your bladder pain to zero, and you will always have to manage it." . . . *Despair.*

Dr. Noblett: "In some people, the bladder pain completely goes away." . . . *Hope!*

Standing on the sidelines watching this rollercoaster of emotion, Alex would say, "Why do you give them so much power?"

Then, one day as I sat in yet another waiting room, I noticed a man sitting next to me with braces on his legs and atrophied hands. I told him I was a physical therapist and asked about his condition.

The man told me he had been completely paralyzed for two years with Guillain-Barré syndrome, an illness that attacks the peripheral nervous system. He'd spent over a decade working to get his strength back, and now he walked short distances with a cane and had limited use of his hands. He told me that when he was at his lowest point, the doctors were about to put him on a respirator to breathe and told him he might not make it. At that point, he realized something: The doctors were giving him their best information based on their experience and what was known at the time, but they were not all-knowing. They didn't know what he was experiencing inside, in his heart and mind. From that point on, he started to listen to himself, too.

After hearing his story, I thought, *If I keep some of my own power, I can slow down this emotional rollercoaster.*

Patient Care Dynamics

Over the years, my personal growth changed what I brought to the treatment table and altered the patient care dynamics I experienced.

Pressure to Please

In the beginning when I didn't seem to be progressing, I felt like I was letting down my caregivers. This feeling brought back memories of working with one of my former physical therapy clients, Lola, a seventy-year-old who had suffered a brain injury from a fall in her bathroom. Before my pain began, I visited her home every week to help her learn to walk more normally again. She would often tell me she was worried that she'd perform poorly and disappoint me. Back then, I couldn't understand what she was talking about.

I told Dr. Ryan about feeling pressure to improve so that I could please my caregivers.

"Do you remember when you were working with patients and some would get better and some you could take only so far?" she asked. "When one of your patients didn't do well, you were never mad or disappointed with them. You just wanted the best for them."

That was true. But I also remembered my excitement when Lola improved and the happiness I'd felt knowing I was making a difference in someone's life.

As a patient, I knew that several of my caregivers were invested in me, and when I improved, they felt good and felt a sense of achievement, too. Sometimes, I just wanted to give this gift to them to reciprocate their kind efforts. On some level, I also wanted them to be excited and interested in my case, so they would keep working with me.

Now, after five years of healing, I understand the patient-care dynamic at a deeper level. Wanting to please my caregivers was a reflection of my lack of confidence at the start of this journey. Just like Lola, I felt like I needed to be perfect in order to be accepted, even in a therapeutic environment in which I was paying for the services. Now that I have more inner strength, I am less afraid to fail and to be vulnerable.

As a caregiver, I may have contributed to the pressure to achieve that Lola felt. Whenever we worked together, she would thank me profusely and praise my therapy skills.

One day I replied, "I feel like I've been walking in the desert for a really long time, and working with you is like drinking a glass of water."

I didn't realize how accurate this analogy was until years later. Before my pain, I was depleted internally, and I used my interaction with Lola to fill up. When I was working with patients, many would become attached to me, and this made me feel needed, valuable, and loved. Now, I understand that this subtle co-dependence between caregiver and patient is not optimal for healing.

Over the years, I began to appreciate that my best caregivers were competent in their skills and also solidly confident. They worked hard to encourage my healing, but they didn't need me to get better to meet their goals or to fill their needs. Because they were emotionally healthy, they could focus more powerfully on my healing.

As I grew personally through these painful years, I started to move from co-dependence to independence in all of my relationships. This also changed how I worked with clients.

The Healing Spark

When I was teaching courses on how to rehabilitate patients with neurological disorders, I always ended the year by saying, "It is important to have knowledge and skills. If you were my physical therapist, I would definitely want you to know what you were doing. But it is also crucial to connect with your patients and treat them with compassion. What you do is important, but who you are makes all the difference."

At the time, this was a nice sentiment and a good way to end the course. But now, after being a patient for so long, I have directly experienced the power of those words.

When I look back over my five-and-a-half-year journey with pain, it is clear that I've had the best outcomes with caregivers who were not only competent but also peaceful and grounded. If a caregiver is solidly focused on my well-being, it helps to unlock my body's healing potential. I can more effectively use what they have to offer for my healing. This is true across the board, with all types of doctors, therapists, and alternative-medicine practitioners. When my caregiver has an abundant spirit, I can use a spark of it to jumpstart my healing.

Getting Attached

From the very beginning, I formed emotional attachments to my caregivers. I was in a painful and difficult spot, and they were my hope for a better life. For the first few years of my illness, I wanted to have a personal connection with each of my caregivers; I felt it was important for my healing. Sometimes, I thought of my caregivers as my friends or family. I had to remind myself that we never met outside of the clinic and that I didn't have to pay my friends to spend time with me.

Several years later, Iben, my life coach, told me that clients often become emotionally attached to their caregivers. She said that for many people, working with a caregiver (either on a physical or emotional level) is the first time in their life they have really felt accepted and cared for.

One of the best examples of this attachment came at the end of my first course of physical therapy with Julie. We had worked together for eighteen months, and my muscle spasms were at a low enough level that I could manage the condition myself. As I was leaving the room at the end of my last treatment session, I burst out crying. My emotions both surprised and embarrassed me. I felt especially connected with Julie. She knew all the intricacies of my care and often took on the role of case manager, all the while helping to hold me together emotionally. My tears were a sign of my gratitude for her skilled treatments and guidance as well as a reflection of my fear of leaving the safety net of her care.

Developing close connections with my caregivers helped to heal some of the emotional contributions to my pelvic pain. These relationships helped to build my confidence and encouraged me to be authentically myself.

However, there is a risk of linking all this positive interaction with being sick, and I didn't want to get stuck in the patient role in order to feel loved. So, in order to fully heal, I had to take this newfound sense of worth and use it to develop relationships outside of the therapy environment. Over time, I weaned off the support of my caregivers and developed my own loving connections.

About four and a half years into my illness, while I was working with Karen Axelrod using the CranioSacral approach, I recognized that our relationship was different. Even though she was very kind, she was detached from me on a personal level, and this was fine with me. After years of healing, I had developed my own internal resources and external support system, so I could focus on my healing rather than on the connection between us.

Becoming Autonomous

My best caregivers have been those who easily adapted to my changing needs, held my hand when I needed it, and encouraged my independence as I healed. Over those five years of treatment, I gradually transitioned from passively accepting support and guidance to actively choosing and directing my care. Here are a few examples of this change:

During my initial physical therapy treatments, Julie skillfully worked with my body while providing emotional support and guidance on how to manage the condition. Now when I work in physical therapy with Nicole, we collaborate throughout the session, telling each other how my body is responding from our different perspectives and deciding together how the treatment should proceed.

In the beginning, Dr. Ryan prescribed medication, referred me to other medical services, and gave me guidance and emotional support. Over time, we began working as partners to manage my condition. She continued to give me advice, and I often told her about treatments I'd adopted and new discoveries I'd made. As an example of this collaboration, almost five years into my illness, I told Dr. Ryan that I had an intuitive sense I no longer needed my pain medication, Cymbalta. She reviewed the status of my condition, confirmed that it was important to listen to my body's wisdom, and gave me instructions on how to wean off the medication.

About the time I stopped taking Cymbalta, Dr. Ryan retired from her medical practice, challenging my sense of autonomy. In years past, losing her as a physician would have sent me into a panic, but now I was calm because I knew I had the personal resources and professional support I needed to manage my condition.

5

Managing the Mind

Until I experienced prolonged pain myself, I'd never appreciated how difficult it was to live with. In this chapter I share some of the mental challenges I faced during the first year and the actions, advice, and encouragement that helped get me through. If you are suffering with chronic pain, hearing about my experience may help you feel less alone, and if you are in a similar state of mind, perhaps the advice that was helpful for me will also give you hope. If you have not experienced the challenge of prolonged pain, I hope these descriptions will help you to empathize with those who carry this burden.

Psychotherapy

At the very start of the pain, my friend Carolyn, who is a physician, suggested I talk with a therapist to help myself and to lighten the emotional load on my family. Dr. Ryan explained that chronic pain could decrease the serotonin levels in the brain, which can lead to depression. So, not only was I dealing with depressing stuff, but my body was also being set up for depression neurobiologically. Going to therapy was easier to accept because I initiated it myself and my initial focus was on helping my family cope with the illness. When I began counseling, I had no idea the support and guidance I received would be so helpful and crucial to my recovery.

I found psychotherapy to be helpful for many reasons. During my counseling sessions, my psychologist, Jackie, gave me strategies to help stave off depression and adjust to the changes in my life and the loss that surrounded the illness. During that first painful year, I had lost a lot: my father, my job, my sense of extended family, and my health. When other people in my life were afraid, overwhelmed, or simply not interested enough to talk, Jackie was there.

Just like everyone on the planet, I carried around my own set of negative thoughts, issues, and fears. But when I was in pain, carrying this old stuff was more difficult, and the pain brought a whole new set of baggage to carry. Jackie helped me to uncover some of these issues, and that helped to lighten my load.

On one of my first visits with Dr. Chalfin, he told me, "I'm glad you are seeing a psychologist. These chronic conditions are really tough." He was right. Living with chronic pain requires great mental fortitude.

Journaling

From the beginning of my illness, it seemed like everyone was encouraging me to write, from friends to caregivers to strangers. When the pain first began, I ran into an acquaintance of mine in the gym locker room. We saw each other around town about once a year, and every time we met we would rapidly share at a deep level. We are not part of each other's daily lives, but we have always felt oddly connected. So that day in the locker room I told her all about my pain.

After listening intently she looked into my eyes and said, "You should write." She told me she had recently started journaling herself and found that writing was a window into her mind.

So I began to write. I found that letting the journal page carry my thoughts really helped to lighten my overall burden. Once my issues and fears had a chance to settle outside of my spinning mind, they were often clearer and easier to deal with. Writing allowed me to appreciate where I've been and to see the growth that accompanied the pain. When I was feeling discouraged, it was helpful to have some measure that I was actually moving forward in the chaos.

Some of the best advice I received came from my own journal page. One night about nine months into my pain, I wrote in my journal quickly and spontaneously, and the words that spilled out gave me great encouragement:

I just want to run and get away from this pain; it is driving me crazy!
Be quiet; be with it; it is still a part of you.
Do all you can to maximize your healing.
Ride it out, and be present with the experience.
Love yourself through it.
Peace will creep in; it will seep around the borders of your softening
resistance.

I used my journal in two different ways during this journey. Early in my illness, my journal was my friend to whom I poured out my heart. This book contains many "discussions" with my inner self during my first two and a half years of pain.

Later, when I began to work with my life coach, Iben, my journaling style changed. Throughout the week prior to each meeting, I would document my experiences, thoughts, and emotions in short phrases, and then I would use these notes to guide our sharing during my session. After each meeting, I would record what Iben had said and what I'd learned. Writing kept me engaged in the healing process and advanced my insight.

This process was so helpful that I continued it even when I wasn't seeing Iben. About once a month I summarized these notes into a narrative form, which eventually became the second part of this book.

Thoughts in the Dark

The pain I experienced during the roughest parts of my journey was at the ideal level for me to give a voice to the mental challenges of chronic pain. I suffered enough to appreciate how it feels to fall into despair, but I wasn't too debilitated to write about it. Many people are suffering at a much higher level than me. I hope this section gives a little voice to their pain and a bit of credibility to their experience.

Catastrophic Thinking

In the very beginning when Dr. Chalfin (my urologist) picked up on my anxious worry, he told me I couldn't fix my physical condition by thinking about it, and he encouraged me to be easy on myself. But how could I not think about it? How could I not be anxious? The pain was intense and relentless, and my doctors didn't know a whole lot about what was causing it or what my outcome would be. With all that uncertainty, I filled in the gaps with worst-case scenarios. I pictured myself never being able to leave the house; going to the bathroom every fifteen minutes, day and night; being wracked with pain 24/7; and being unlovable and lonely. Such catastrophic thinking was seductive, but once activated, it only amplified my suffering.

Stressing about these envisioned negative outcomes and feeling helpless to do anything to prevent them from happening caused me great mental anguish. That, in turn, ramped up the stress response within my body—the exact opposite of the inner calm needed to promote healing. It sapped me of the energy I needed to deal with the present moment, and it drained those around me, too. My husband, Alex, told me that he could handle what was happening now, but when I piled on the future, it was just too much for him. He said he wanted to be there for me no matter what happened, but if I burned him out worrying about the future, he might be too tired or sick to help me when I really needed it.

During that dark period of my life, a newsletter from my husband's work place came to the house, in which I found the following two quotes that seemed to speak directly to me:

"The best thing about the future is that it only comes one day at a time."

— Abraham Lincoln

"Do not anticipate trouble or worry about what may never happen. Keep in the sunlight."

— Benjamin Franklin

I started to realize that the past and future were in my mind and that the only reality was the present moment, the here and now. When I didn't pile on fears of the future, getting through the present difficulty became surprisingly easier. Because I only had power to act in the present moment, that was the best, and really, the only way to influence my future.

Years later, my life coach, Iben, told me that people fall into despair when they don't think there is anything they can do about their pain. She is right. When I started to find more ways to help myself during the fourth month of pain, I felt a glimmer of hope and my mental anguish began to subside.

Hiding the Pain

At the beginning of each psychotherapy session with Jackie, she would always ask me what my pain level was that day. Most of the time I would say it was about a three. She would usually tell me she could see me and the pain was obviously greater than a level three. She told me when her bladder was hurting, that particular kind of pain was always at least a level six, and it made her feel like she was going crazy.

Jackie encouraged me not to ignore my pain and to be honest about my pain level. She said, "I know you are just trying to get on with your life, but the pain is here now."

How right she was, as this entry from my journal indicates:

I am in a very lonely place, and I deny my pain because I want out of here. I am a contortionist trying all positions to hide my pain and make it okay.

The Deep, Dark Hole

As the weeks and months of pain wore on, I felt like I'd fallen into a deep, dark abyss. I started to lose hope that I'd ever get out of there.

My journal entry from this time shows how trapped I felt:

I feel like I'm in a dark hole and I can't get out. I'm trying to see the sun. But the hole keeps reminding me how deep it really is.

I repeated this sentiment to my psychologist, Jackie, during my next counseling session. She acknowledged I was truly in a hole but suggested that I alter my mental image a bit to help myself move forward. She had me imagine a hole with beautiful green, marble walls and a soft surface upon which I could sit. She said sometimes I would have to just sit down there and rest. Then, she had me picture rope ladders hanging down the sides of the hole. The ladders represented ways I would find to alleviate the pain, like yoga and physical therapy. She said that, over time, I would find even more ladders to help me climb out of that hole.

Over the years, I pulled down a lot of ladders with initial skepticism and warily stepped up on them. Some took me nowhere, but others supported my weight and helped me to climb part way out of my hole of suffering. No one ladder scaled the whole distance, but different ones were effective at different points of the ascent.

This was the first time a therapist used guided visual imagery with me. Even though the picture gave me some hope, I didn't revisit this image after my counseling session.

Years later, I would use visual imagery again with my life coach, Iben, and as part of two different alternative approaches: Myofascial Release and CranioSacral therapy. Unlike my sessions with Jackie, in this work the internal images were self-created and linked to my body sensations. These internal images often contained major information about the mental and emotional issues that were entwined with my physical pain.

Over the years, the use of imagery would be crucial to developing my awareness of the mind-body connection and to my recovery. This was one of the most surprising ladders I eventually pulled down to ascend out of that pit of pain!

Releasing Emotion

Four months into my pain, my then thirteen-year-old son, Alex, and I were sitting in church, and the congregation began saying a prayer for people in pain—and the tears began flowing down my cheeks. Try as I might, I just couldn't make them stop. My son stiffened and tried to keep his composure. When I asked him to get me some tissues, he practically bolted down the aisle, clearly relieved to get out of there. A few minutes later when the congregation began to sing my deceased mother's favorite song, "On Eagle's Wings," I rushed out of the chapel and into the bathroom, locked myself in a stall, leaned my head against the wall, and sobbed.

At my next counseling appointment, I asked Jackie, "Do you think I am slipping into depression?"

She asked me if I cried during my everyday tasks, like taking my kids to school. I told her it only happened when I was alone and on that day in church. She told me I would have times and maybe days when I broke down, but then I'd rally again. This was normal, she assured me.

This was my first experience of an emotional release, and I would understand later why this situation triggered the response. Over the years, I would have many situations that triggered an emotional release like this one, and they often gave me clues about a mental, emotional, or spiritual issue that was coming to the surface to be healed.

At the beginning of my illness, I rarely expressed emotion, so to have it burst out without my control was embarrassing, and I wondered about my mental health. But, in time, I realized that holding my emotions inside was the unhealthy approach.

Over the years, I learned that I wasn't weak; in fact, I had tried to stay strong for too long. I wasn't overly emotional, as I'd thought. In fact, I was the opposite; I was holding myself with a steely resolve and not allowing myself to feel. Having an emotional release wasn't a sign that I was breaking down; it was a signal that I was finally opening up. It wasn't a sign that I couldn't handle my life; it was a signal that I was ready to start experiencing my life.

Impermanence

My friend Lisa is also a physical therapist. When my husband was in Europe and my suffering was at its peak, I invited her over for lunch. I was in major pain and major denial, and I couldn't eat.

Lisa looked at me over the table with concern and said, "It won't always be this bad. Your pain will improve, and if it doesn't fully resolve, you will learn how to cope with it better." My pain and anxiety were too great to focus on anything Lisa said. Even though I wrote her comment in my journal that night, it didn't really sink in.

My second lesson in the possibility of impermanence came six months later as I waited for yet another appointment. I sat in a sandwich shop sipping my soup and watching the long line of customers streaming past my table. Most were talking casually with their co-workers about things like work projects, fashion, and movies. I felt heavy and separated from their world, and I wondered if I would ever be there again.

When I shared those thoughts and feelings with Jackie, she told me, "Don't worry, you won't always be in this dark place."

Really? I thought. *I won't always be suffering?* That was a novel concept to me, because at the time, I thought the pain would never end. On that day, Jackie opened a window and let in some light.

As Alex and I were walking one evening about eight months into the pain, I told him I was discouraged and wondered whether I would ever get better. He said he was sure I was going to improve but didn't know when it was going to happen. Then, he told me about a book he had read about prisoners of war. He said the POWs who wanted to be free by a certain holiday or year would become depressed when the date passed and they weren't released. The POWs who did the best mentally believed they would be freed someday but didn't set a specific time for when it had to happen.

Flaring Up

The pain would wax and wane, taking my emotions along for the ride. When the pain levels dropped, I would feel elated, only to fall into despair when the pain reared up again.

My physical therapist, Julie, would encourage me to try to keep my emotions on an even keel and to ride it out when the pain flared up. But that was really difficult to do.

The following excerpts from my journal reflect my thoughts about the flare-ups over the first year and the encouragement that helped me get through:

Well, I've been flared up for the past four days. I can handle it better now. I try to focus on the facts and not all the scary thoughts and dark emotions that the pain brings. It's like my pain and I are in a relationship, and it's best if I don't remember our past history or worry about a future together. It helps when I just focus on the present. But sometimes it gets to me, and last night when everyone was asleep, I just sat in the dark living room and cried for a long time. I guess being honest with my emotions is handling it, too.

I have aches and a burning pain that I haven't felt for months, so to have it return is so scary and disheartening. The actual pain is much less than I've experienced before, but I am just so full of dealing with it that now smaller amounts of pain quickly fill me to overflowing. The pain is less, but it bugs me more! I used to be so happy for small windows in my day that had less pain or no pain. But now when I'm hurting, it makes me mad because I know what it is like to be pain-free.

Julie explained that my baseline had switched from pain to pain-free, and this was a sign of progress. She told me I was not alone and most of her patients got mad at this stage.

I was flared up over the last few weeks. My thoughts were racing, and I got really active. Spinning like this was my way of trying to get away from the pain, but it just made it worse. In all that frantic activity, I actually pulled away from Alex and the kids, and I felt so lonely.

Next time, I'll try to slow down. I'll meditate more, and I'll step toward my family to get support. I'll try to remember that I can't hide from the fear and discomfort. I have to be brave enough to go right into it and accept it with loving-kindness. This doesn't mean I have to like it or want it. I'm definitely not happy about it! But just accepting it as part of my experience may help me be more at peace within the pain.

It is the one-year anniversary of this pain, and I have been flared up for the past week. On my way to physical therapy, the tears flowed down my cheeks, over my chin, and into my lap for the entire thirty-minute drive. When I entered the clinic, the tears would not stop, and this was embarrassing!

Julie told me not to worry, that a lot of tears had been shed on her treatment table. She told me the body remembers, and many of her patients could attribute their flare-ups to really emotional times in their lives. She thought my current flare-up was related to the trauma I'd experienced when my pain first began.

She hugged me and told me she was sorry I was hurting and she knew I would be better. She described the worst-case scenario for my level of healing and helped me see that as manageable. Then, she encouraged me to trust my caregivers and to stay calm. That day, she lifted me out of despair by giving me compassion, hope, support, and a plan. Bless her loving heart.

My Thoughts, My Reality?

During one of my first counseling sessions, Jackie warned me that when you have an illness, especially one people aren't familiar with, you will get all types of unsolicited advice. The very next day, I had that exact experience.

It was the third month of pain, and I was sitting in the whirlpool at the gym. The topic of conversation turned once again to a litany of everyone's injuries and illnesses. After hearing only a little about my condition, a fat guy with an English accent told me that I'd asked the Universe for my pain and brought it on myself. He said I should be a more positive person. I told him my mother was one of the most positive people you could meet, but she'd died from ALS, just like my grandmother. I argued that there are genetic predispositions for different illnesses. He replied that my mom probably had a fearful thought about ALS at one point in her life, and that's why she got it. Although my response was polite and calm, internally I was devastated.

Only in my journal did I express my true feelings:

Talk about blaming the victim! What crazy person would ever wish this pain on themselves! It also brings shame that you screwed up—made a mess of things and now you may not be able to be healed. And if there is some truth to what this guy said, what else have I asked for?

On my next appointment with my acupuncturist, Pam, I told her that the idea of having somehow created my reality with my own thoughts was really tough to accept now that I had so much pain and didn't know if I'd get getter. She reassured me that conscious thoughts didn't automatically create my reality; it wasn't that simple.

But I knew my attitude could affect my healing, and I wanted to cover my bases just in case there was any truth to this guy's idea. So I wrote the following plan in my journal:

I have a choice in how I view what I've been handed. If being positive can, in any way, make positive things happen, I want to take advantage of this for my own healing! So, from this point forward, I will turn my thoughts to healing and set my mind on full recovery. But I won't put pressure on myself that it has to turn out this way. I will think about the factors that contributed to my loss of health, and I will change all of them that are in my control. But I won't spend time feeling guilty about the past or blaming myself for my illness. I will consider this illness a learning experience for my soul and grab all the good lessons I can. I will use this theory to move forward by accepting the responsibility but not the guilt.

Over the years, many theories came my way about the relationship between my thoughts, emotions, and life experiences. But more powerful for me than those ideas was my direct experience. I found that when I became consciously aware of the patterns in my life and the long-held beliefs I had previously carried at a subconscious level, I could change them. Over time, I uncovered the constricting, fear-based patterns, ideas, and emotions that I carried. Once I recognized them, I could choose to replace them with more expanding, loving options. For me, this process was crucial to healing physically as well as mentally, emotionally, and spiritually. This work also led to dramatic positive changes in my life. In the next section of this book I share my experience with this process of uncovering the layers of thought, emotion, and behavior and healing them.

Making a Mental Plan

After a full year of pain, I began trying to manage my own mind, as evidenced by this journal entry:

This pain is really a rude guest! It shows up unannounced and often at the worst of times, and I never know how long it is going to stay, disrupting my life. And not only that, this pain often brings its friends: fear, anxiety, and depression.

To cope with these nasty visits, here is my plan:
* *Accept what is, and don't deny the pain.*
* *Do everything in your power to maximize healing.*
* *Be present, and try not to focus on past pain or possible future pain.*

- *Rest, and be kind to yourself when you are hurting.*
- *Let yourself cry or lean when the pain beats you down.*
- *Choose to be peaceful.*
- *Be grateful for the good things of each day.*
- *Cherish the love that flows in your life.*

Gratitude

My massage therapist, Chris, told me that one of the best ways to see your life from a new perspective is to practice being grateful. At first her suggestion made me bristle, because when I was little, my mother often told me to be grateful when I was upset, and so I would shove back negative emotions and force a positive attitude. I knew that this was part of the reason I got sick in the first place, and I no longer wanted to hide my pain.

Throughout my childhood, I thought my mother used the notion of gratitude to deny negative emotions and to avoid dealing with them. As my mother grew during her own illness, she became sincerely grateful even as her body totally failed. On one of my last visits to her home, I arrived from the airport and found her reclining on a padded chaise lounge on her screened-in porch. Taking the seat next to her, I registered the shell of her body, now almost completely paralyzed, her labored breathing, and the subtle tension around her eyes that told me she was in pain.

Then, she smiled at me with sparkling eyes and said, "It is just as I imagined it would be at the end—the breeze, the birds, the music. It's beautiful."

I had carried around quite a bit of resentment and anxiety during my years on this planet prior to my illness, and I might not have chosen an upbeat path through my pain had I been left to my own devices. But I had watched my mother, the Queen of Gratitude, who was a master at focusing on the best and beautiful parts of her life even as she was dying. Those memories encouraged me to look beyond the pain.

When I looked at the whole experience, I could see that, alongside the pain, were goodness and beauty, too. When I turned my focus to the positive parts of my experience, I saw even more things to be grateful for.

When I appreciated the good in my life, my mind was more at ease, and that seemed to calm my nervous system and decrease my pain. Gratitude was healing.

Believing

Eighteen months into my pain, a clear image of the poster that was above my bed throughout my childhood popped into my head. On the black background was a photograph of an ethereal ballerina in the middle of a leap, and underneath the picture was a quote by William Arthur Ward: "If you can imagine it, you can achieve it. If you can dream it, you can become it."

I thought, *I'm going to imagine and dream of being pain-free.*

In my psychotherapist, Jackie's, waiting room is a framed poem, which I read before each visit. It was written by one of her other patients, a woman who clearly understood the dark place I inhabited. Blending her words with my own, I wrote this encouragement for myself:

B Behold the beauty that can be found in even the darkest places.

E Enjoy the clarity of knowing what is most important in life.

L Let yourself cry, and live to laugh again.

I Invite comfort; allow yourself to lean when you need it.

E Envelop yourself in the healing power of love.

V Value the smallest of things, for nothing is insignificant.

E Eve will give way to dawn, and this darkness will turn into light.

6

Seeing in the Dark

Prior to my illness, I never thought about or searched for spiritual truth. But then, through this painful journey, a spiritual side of me that had been buried came alive again. This chapter describes my spiritual state before my illness and chronicles my spiritual experiences from the beginning of my illness, when the pain was at its peak, until two years later, when the levels became less intense.

Before the Pain

One of my last visits with my mother, about five and a half years before my pain began, clearly depicts my spiritual state before this challenging illness.

Over the course of seven years, my mother had gradually become paralyzed as a result of amyotrophic lateral sclerosis (ALS). During what turned out to be the last six months of her life, it was clear she was fading fast, so I traveled every month from Southern California to Chicago to see her. Whenever I arrived from the airport and entered her small ranch home, I'd brace myself for another level of physical decline.

On one such day, I found her in the family room with the sun shining on her still, bony frame, which seemed to be engulfed in the folds of the maroon recliner. I asked her how she spent her days now that she could no longer walk. She motioned to the stack of books beside her and told me that she read inspiring books and spent time thinking and praying.

Then, my mom looked directly at me and said, "You know, Mary Ruth, it's important to take time for spiritual growth."

I didn't say a word, but I remember thinking, *I don't have time for that kind of stuff.* At that point in my life, I thought humans were probably nothing more than the sum of their genes, just playing out the patterns of their inherited biology.

The Big Stick

Some people grow spiritually as their lives challenge them. But until after the pain began when I was in my mid-forties, I'd never embarked on any type of spiritual quest, and the traumas of life had never altered the way I viewed things in any profound or permanent way. That wasn't because I'd lived a perfectly charmed life or because my challenges were light. In fact, my medical history was brimming with past physical challenges.

When I was twenty-five, I injured a disc in my neck while working with a patient. I attended physical therapy for several months and lived with intermittent neck pain for years. My neck pain made it difficult to treat patients on a full-time basis, so I went to graduate school and started to teach.

Katherine was born when I was thirty, and it was a rough ride. I endured twenty-four hours of labor, eclampsia, an emergency Cesarean section, and then, a few days later, double pneumonia, seizures, and a stroke (cortical venous thrombosis). I was in a coma and on a respirator for a week, with my blood pressure soaring, even though I was taking the most potent medications available. Later, Dr. Ryan told me she'd counted five times when they didn't know whether I was going to survive. But I made it through without any lasting deficits.

At age forty, right after my mother died, I ruptured a different disc in my neck. I again diligently attended physical therapy for months, and I narrowly escaped surgery.

Four years later, I went through several more months of physical therapy after a car accident to rehabilitate leg weakness and back pain.

Then, when I was forty-five, I began the long journey with debilitating pelvic pain.

After hearing my medical history, my massage therapist, Chris, said, "When you don't heed the lesson, the stick just keeps getting bigger."

"Well, I'd better get the message this time," I said, "Because that next stick will surely kill me!"

I was like the phoenix that burns up in the fire and keeps coming back again. With each resurrection, though, I returned with the same old baggage. I hadn't even paused for reflection after Katherine's birth became a near-death experience.

But this last challenge was different; it changed me. The intense, chronic pelvic pain was the catalyst I needed to grow, and that fire of suffering transformed me in many ways.

The Night of Darkness and Light

The pelvic pain had been bearing down on me for two months. During that time, I'd traveled throughout Europe, battled a severe bout of the flu, and lost my father. Then, suddenly, for the first time since the pain began, the activity stopped and I was alone. Alex was gone on a two-week business trip in Germany, and I lacked a support network beyond him. The pain rose higher and higher, and it wouldn't let me sleep. I would lie in bed with my pulse pounding in my ears, and when I'd finally doze off, the pain would rouse me from a dead sleep with an intensity that terrified me. I was handling everything I needed to do for my kids by myself, but the pain was taking a toll.

One night, after dropping off Katherine at a friend's house, I stopped at a red light and gazed numbly at a landscape cast only in shades of gray. Sitting there in the car watching the cars go by and the people scurrying about, I felt like I was looking at a world I no longer inhabited. It all seemed superficial and unreal.

That same night, I started reading *The Power of Now*, by Eckhart Tolle. My brother had given me the book one Christmas, and it had been collecting dust on the shelf above my bed for a couple of years. I'd tried reading it once before but didn't get past the introduction, in which the author describes how he came to the realization that he was more than his body and mind. At the time, I'd concluded that the writer, who had suffered severe depression prior to this experience, had diminished activity in the frontal lobes of his brain and activated other parts of his brain in response to this stress. In my view, his new perceptions were neatly categorized but completely suspect, so I'd shut the book. Despite this earlier skepticism, at the end of that dark day during the second month of the pain, I found myself reading *The Power of Now*.

The first chapter discusses the idea that we are more than the activity of our minds. The author invites the reader to tune in to his or her inner dialogue and to recognize that underneath all that chatter there is more. I was well aware of this inner dialogue; mine was incessant and often negative. That night, as I concentrated on moving beneath all that internal noise, I suddenly felt fullness in my heart and an electric wave flow from my heart all the way to my fingers and toes.

The next night, once again, the pain was heavy on me and I lay in bed crying. I called out to my deceased parents, "If there is any way you can help me, now would be a good time." I thought about my dad, and a little tingling went through my body. Then, I thought about my mom, and wave after wave of electric energy passed from the top of my head through my body and out my fingers and toes. After the fifth time, I started to laugh and said out loud, "Okay, okay! I get that you loved me."

In the past, I would have written off these experiences as a neural pathway in overdrive because of the pain. But it was different this time. I just knew that even if my body were consumed with pain and illness and even if my mind suffered from major depression, a deeper part of me, my spirit, would never die. In that moment, I also knew that when I felt I had nowhere else to turn, there was always more within.

Analyzing the Unknown

That night, a scary experience turned into something exciting, and my predictable life turned into a journey full of potential. At the time, I had no explanation for what had happened to me and why it had changed my perspective, but over the next few months, some information came my way that helped me to accept it.

A week after I started reading *The Power of Now*, I met Myra in the whirlpool at the gym, where, as usual, the topic of conversation was everyone's aches and pains. She talked about living with fibromyalgia and how, after being bedridden for two years, she had rallied over the past year to get her life back. As we walked into the locker room, Myra told me she relied on her connection with God to give her strength. I told her about the night I'd starting reading Tolle's book, what I'd experienced afterward, and how it had made me realize I was more than my body and mind.

"That was the grace of God," Myra said.

That evening, I read these words in *The Power of Now*:

"Awakening is a shift in consciousness in which thinking and awareness separate. . . . The initiation of the awakening process is an act of grace."

A few months later, I read something written by Deepak Chopra that resonated with me. He described how the experience of reality is determined, in part, by one's capability to perceive and process sensory information. Throughout history, the view of reality has changed whenever humans have enhanced their sensory capabilities with technology. For example, before the invention of microscopes and Geiger counters, cells and radiation were unknown to us but always there. Only when these devices enabled us to "perceive" cells and radiation did they become part of our world view. After my experiences on that desperate night, I was more open to the possibility that there is much more in this world than I can pick up with my five senses.

I also thought that my perception of reality could change if my brain were to process the sensory information it received in a different way or with different neural pathways. From my past studies, I knew that much of the brain was uncharted territory, where its function was unknown. I also knew that, with practice and experience, the brain could remodel its structure. I wondered if the stress of that night opened up a latent capability in my brain to process just a bit more of what is already out there.

On a walk in the neighborhood around that time, I mentioned to Alex, "The stars are really out tonight." Suddenly, I realized the silliness of that common statement. The stars are always there, even in the light of day, but now that conditions had changed, I could perceive them.

What had happened to me on that painful night was a little like stargazing. Maybe because it was really, really dark, I could see more.

Low Tide

While sitting and waiting for a physical therapy appointment with Julie, I read in a book that life flows out and recedes, much like the tide. In times of low tide, such as aging and illness, the body and the sense of self diminish. This can create suffering, and one can become defeated by the sense of loss. But there is a positive side to this dynamic, too, for when the ego retreats, it creates space where the spirit can then develop and shine.

I don't remember exactly where I read this, but the message struck a chord with me. I realized there was more than just loss here; there was also potential to grow. Perhaps, through this experience, I might actually be fulfilling the purpose of my soul.

Being Alone

Before my pelvic pain began, being alone rarely felt restful or restorative. When I was by myself, I kept busy with mental or physical tasks and filled the quiet space with talk radio, music, or television. Yet, even with these diversions, my mind would often spin.

Two years into my pain, I found the small journal I kept as a teenager. When I read the following poem, written at age thirteen, I realized that my aversion to being alone had started young.

When I'm Alone

I feel the day's failures, anxieties, defeats and small happiness slip through my fingers
When I'm alone
I picture myself in a mirror and seek out my faults in the reflection of the inner me

When I'm alone
I try to find the me under false beings that wake when I'm with various
people and perish to leave me with myself
When I'm alone
Life is very revealing, uncertain and lonely
When I'm alone

Before my pelvic pain, I always chose to be busy and productive, and I allowed no time for quiet introspection. The following poem, which I wrote at age fifteen, shows that part of me knew this frantic pace was not healthy.

Tired and afraid
Sensitive and frustrated.
Excited, worried and pressured
Is bottled-up me.
I'm trying to discover this me under my emotions.
I need a chance to rest a while
To watch and savor my world
For with the frustration, time will slip my life away.

It took me thirty years and major pain before I chose to follow my own angst-ridden teen advice. When the pain descended and pulled me off of my life, I was alone for most of the day and found it difficult to do all the activities that had once served to distract me from my inner turmoil. I was forced to attend to the needs of my body and mind.

About ten months into my illness, my first massage therapist, Mika, gave me the book, *Simple Truths: Clear and Gentle Guidance on the Big Issues in Life*, by Kent Nerburn. The following passage from that book clearly described the challenge I was facing:

"Time alone is the proving ground of the spirit. You quickly find out if you are at peace with yourself or if the meaning of your life is found only in the superficial affairs of the day. If it is in the superficial affairs of the day, time alone will throw you back upon yourself in a way that will make you grow in wisdom and inner strength."

Those words gave me hope that enduring all that alone time served some purpose.

After the pain had pulled me from my life for about a year, I became more accustomed to quiet solitude, as evidenced by my journal entry from that time:

I used to love drama, thrive on its intensity.
Now, it just makes me hurt.
It is quiet—in my life and in my head.

Silence and Spiritual Connection

At the beginning of my illness, I was working with my patient Lola every week to help her learn to walk more normally after having suffered a brain injury. When I told her about my condition and that I could no longer work with her, she was really worried about me. Because I knew she was a devout Christian, I told her this would be my alone time and reassured her that even Jesus had gone into the desert to be alone. This image didn't have much meaning for me, but I thought the analogy would make Lola feel better. She told me I was wrong; Jesus was never alone. God was with him, and God would be with me, too. She added that alone time is really a gift, because sometimes you need to be quiet in order to hear God's voice.

Right about this time, I read two quotes by Kent Nerburn that reinforced the idea that being alone and quiet can be an opportunity for spiritual connection:

"Solitude is a condition of peace that stands in direct opposition to loneliness. Loneliness is like sitting in an empty room and being aware of the space around you. It is a condition of separateness. Solitude is becoming one with the space around you. It is a condition of union."

"Most people fear being alone because they understand only loneliness. Their understanding begins at the self, and they are comfortable only as long as they are at the center of their understanding. Solitude is about getting the 'I' out of the center of our thoughts so that other parts of life can be experienced in their fullness. It is about abandoning the self as the focus of understanding, and giving ourselves over to the great flowing fabric of the universe."

Living in the Now

When my friend Sandy took me to a yoga class, one year into my pain, I had no idea it would have anything to do with the healing of my spirit. My only hope was that it might ease the pain a little bit or at least distract me from it.

The yoga class combined meditative readings with long-held poses that stretched out the hips and pelvic area. Before class, I told the instructor that I had been dealing with pelvic pain for the past year, so I might not be able to get into all of the poses and would probably have to get up to use the bathroom during class. The instructor told me that was fine and I was probably in an advanced stage of practice already. She said that living with profound pain is considered a gift, an opportunity for spiritual growth. I certainly didn't think of it as a gift! But I noticed that when she gave verbal cues for people to quiet their minds and to focus on the sensations of the body and breath, I didn't need them. Calming my mind was how I had survived the past year of pain.

Later, my acupuncturist, Pam, told me, "Pain forces you to be in the present, or the Now."

She was right. My pain often made me just stop and attend to what was happening with my body. It also sapped me of energy, leaving me with few resources to ruminate about the past or worry about the future.

This was quite a feat, because before the illness, I'd prided myself on having a very active mind that just didn't stop. I was the queen of worry, and I revisited and catalogued every event, every relationship, and every hurt of the past. But after doing some reading, I realized that when I was thinking of the past or future, I was really just revisiting the perception of my life created in my mind. When I wasn't stuck in those backward- or forward-looking thoughts and, instead, focused on now, I was actually interacting with the world.

In other words, I was living. And when my mind was fully in the moment, I found peace.

Listening in the Silence

When my mind wasn't spinning, I began to appreciate the healing messages that were coming at me from all directions in my life.

Expectations and Suffering

I was looking for fabric in a store when a beautiful and very pregnant young woman started flipping through the samples next to me. Our conversation turned from our projects to our lives, and I told her about my disappointment that my extended family had not supported me during my illness.

I had my back to her when she said, "Well, now that you know, you can manage your expectations."

Her words pierced me like an arrow, and I thought, *Oh, that one was meant for me.*

The next day before yoga class, a woman confided that she was hurt by the minimal efforts her daughter made to connect with her. I shared my resentment that my brothers and sisters had not contacted me throughout my illness.

Then, she said, "I heard something yesterday that made a lot of sense: We all want love from certain sources, and it's usually from people who can't give it to us. There is love all around if we are just open to it. And if that isn't enough, getting it from the people we've chosen won't fill us up, either."

That night I read these words of Eckhart Tolle:

"We can place unreasonable demands on the world: Fulfill me, make me happy, make me feel safe, tell me who I am. The world cannot give you those things, and when you no longer have those expectations, all self-created suffering comes to an end."

Ancient Support

One day about eighteen months into my illness, the pain was really flaring up, and I accidentally arrived two hours early for my scheduled physical therapy appointment. To pass the time, I walked over to the Crystal

Cathedral (now Christ Cathedral), an impressive church surrounded by expansive grounds. The weather reflected my mood: cold, drizzly, and overcast.

As I walked the grounds with my head down, I began reading the bible passages that were etched into the path. There, below my feet, lay the words that kept me walking that day:

"Be joyful in hope, patient in affliction, faithful in prayer."

— Romans 12:12

"Do not neglect the gift that is in you."

— Timothy 4:14

"If you can believe all things are possible."

— Mark 9:23

"For God has not given us a spirit of fear, but of power and of love and of a sound mind."

— 2 Timothy 1:7

"Love bears all things, believes all things, hopes all things, endures all things."

— I Corinthians 13:4–7

My Words, My Wisdom

On two dark nights, I wrote down my thoughts as quickly as they came. When I read them later, I wondered where these ideas had come from, because at the time they were written, the words were a stark contrast to the normal ramblings of my conscious mind.

Here are those words that jumped off the page of my journal and into my heart:

No one cares about me. I have no friends, and I am all alone.
   You are never alone.
I need to entertain and achieve in order to be accepted and loved.
   You are loveable and valuable just as you are.
I need people to understand and like me.

Not everyone will get you and it's not your responsibility to fix it.
Drama and intensity are necessary and invigorating.
   Life can be easy and not boring.
I'm afraid of what is next if I give this up.
   It will all be okay, trust me. I am with you on this journey.
If I have control over this, what if I don't do it right and I fail? What if I never get better?
   You are healing. Be patient; you are just not there yet.

Loving Myself

When I described my life in my teenage journal, it was clear I was being blown around like a young sapling, my sense of worth wildly fluctuating with the words and actions of others.

One of the poems I found, written at age eighteen, clearly depicts my insecurity and search for approval.

Soft, flowing motions of fantasy expression flow with the music
On pretended studio floor
Lightly leaping and landing to the music of life
Searching in the blur of the audience for subtle applause
My inner being pushes enthusiastically into position and interpretations
   of my experience
As the applause quiets, the wonder of graceful liquid movement is
   interrupted
By the dancer's self doubt.

Aging hadn't healed this fundamental concern that I was unlovable. As an adult I still looked for validation in the faces of those around me.

On one of my first visits, Jackie told me people kept telling me wonderful things about myself but I didn't take them in. She said, "You have a hole in your cup."

I also remembered my first Reiki session with Stella. I was lying face-down on a blanket in my living room in tears. She asked me to think of all the ways I'd showed love to my family that morning, even the little things. I thought of the touches, the words, the lunches, and the drive with the kids. Then, Stella told me to pull all that love back to myself. She said I needed to love myself, all parts of me.

I started to realize that I needed to be kind to myself when I was in pain and that I was the only one who could love myself through it.

My journal entry one year into my pain shows this new perspective:

I am kinder to myself now. I noticed it the other day when I looked in the mirror. Instead of focusing on my age spots, wrinkles, and gray hair, I thought, Look at you—a vibrant, aging woman! Now, I can hear my friends being tough on themselves, not giving themselves credit, driving themselves, and I think, Oh, I was there, too.

A little memory popped into my head this week. It was Saturday night, right after bath time, and a girl of four danced around her living room in a white little slip, her wet hair in pin curls. She was pretending to be a fairy. Welcome back, little me! I see you, and I will be kind to you now. It is safe.

Inner Strength

After being in pain for about a year, I began to look within for strength to heal. Two journal entries from this time depict this switch in my perspective:

This is my journey, and I'm alone in it. This doesn't mean I'm abandoned; Alex helps me often. It is just that I need to become my own best friend. I am beginning to find my own spiritual strength to come to grips with this oh-so-difficult journey. Like Eckhart Tolle's analogy of a beggar sitting on a box of gold, I have to believe that everything I need to handle it is already within me. I was always looking outside for validation and strength. Now, I need to look further within.

To maintain my sanity with this pain, I had to dig deeper, and there I have found a glimmer of my internal strength and light. I am becoming more grounded now, and my sense of self doesn't fully rely on the perceptions of others. It is time for me to heal myself, to fill from within, and to move on to the rest of my life.

A few weeks after the second entry, above, Jackie and I were finishing up a counseling session, and she said, "I'm afraid you'll think it is strange to say this, but it's like when you feel it in your gut—a negative feeling just being next to someone. But in this case, it's the opposite feeling, and this kind of positive energy is not common here because of the work I do. Instead of your energy being scattered all around you, it is centered within you and strong. You seem to be really present."

I told her I had found a new book that had been collecting dust on my shelf for a couple years—*A New Earth*, the second Eckhart Tolle book my brother had given me. While reading the book over that past week, I'd felt a strange kind of fullness, like an energy flowing throughout my body.

Jackie asked me whether Alex had noticed this energy emanating from me, too. So that night on our walk I asked him.

He said, "That is a good description of it. Two weeks ago, you were getting stronger, and then the pain returned and you lost some of that power. But the last two days that centered strength is back."

Nurtured by Nature

One day while watching the birds in my backyard, I remembered sitting with my mother in her kitchen after she'd been living with ALS for several years. She was looking out the window at the birds in her own backyard when she said, "It's strange, but I feel so connected to nature now. Like it is a part of me and I am a part of it."

When my pain set in, I began to more fully appreciate those words she'd shared with me so many years before.

My connection with nature began three months into my illness as I sat in yet another waiting room, heavy with pain. The same thoughts were repeating over and over in my head: *The life you knew is over. You will never be able to work or be productive again.* Then, I remembered Eckhart Tolle's encouragement to attend to what is around you at the moment. The red mums sitting on the glass table in front of me leapt into my view. They were bathed in sunlight and surrounded by baby's breath, and their delicate petals stood shoulder to shoulder in concentric circles, with the tiniest ones in the center and each row to the outside having petals just a little bit larger. My tears blurred the image, and I realized that during that moment, nature had whisked me away from my painful body and my spinning mind.

After this experience, nature started to greet me in the midst of suburbia. Following are my fondest memories of this newfound relationship with the natural world:

In winter, as I walked barefoot on the cold, wet sand of the Pacific Ocean, the waves rolled toward me, their crests reflecting the full white moon shining overhead like a beacon in the black sky.

In spring, as I strolled with Alex in our neighborhood each night, the green buds, fluffy leaves, and flowers put on an art show.

In summer, the waves rose up in a thunderous symphony as I watched Katherine run down the beach to place a rescued starfish on the jetty rocks.

In fall, Alex stoked the bonfire and I stood behind him, resting my head on his back, as the golden sunset silhouetted the kids racing down the beach. The rain clouds, a fluffy blanket over our heads, lightly sprinkled our faces, and behind us a full rainbow arched over the wetlands.

Nature's show was sometimes simple and sometimes spectacular, but always a gift. When I was centered and peaceful, I was more aware of nature; when I was aware of nature, I became more centered and peaceful. Over time, my connection with nature became a barometer for my connection with my soul. Over the years, this relationship between the natural world and my spirit continued to mature and deepen.

Growing Deep Roots

In the middle of my second year of pain, I was heading toward the elevator after a physical therapy appointment with Julie when a tall, blonde woman about my age emerged from another office and strode toward me. As we neared the elevator, she lifted up a chocolate truffle and teased, "Don't you wish you had one of these?" I held out the peppermint in my hand and laughed, telling her I felt somewhat cheated. She told me that to get the chocolate you had to be a cancer patient, so I probably wouldn't want it. Then, I told her that to get the peppermint you had to be a patient with chronic pelvic pain.

After this introduction, the two of us stood outside the medical building doors for two hours sharing our separate journeys. Catherine was proactive, positive, and radiant, and she had lived with stage-four cancer for ten years. When I told her that throughout my whole experience I'd felt supported by nature, she nodded in agreement. Then, at the same time, we said, "Especially trees."

Catherine looked around and in a hushed tone said, "I haven't told anyone this yet, for fear they would think I was crazy, but I think you'll understand: A tree once talked to me. Not actual talking, but while I was looking at it, a voice in my head said, 'Grow your roots very, very deep and hold on. There are big storms coming in your life. You will bend, but will not break.'"

This Too Shall Pass

During the second year of pain, I noticed that—just as the trees, flowers, air, and birds all changed with the seasons—so, too, did my body have its own cyclical rhythm, changing with the day, the week, the month, the season, and the year. Even my pain and emotions cycled up and down.

About the time I started to appreciate the cyclical nature of life, I read a section in *A New Earth* in which Tolle discusses the spiritual significance of the adage, *This too shall pass*. I laughed out loud when I read those words, because that exact phrase was my mother's mantra. I used to get mad when she said it, thinking it was just her way of ignoring and discounting the pain of a difficult situation.

Eckhart explains that these four simple words point to an acceptance of and a peace with the fact that change is constant in life and nothing stays the same. I realized that, toward the end of her life, my mother understood this deeper meaning of the old saying. She exuded acceptance and peace even as her muscles got progressively weaker and her ability to function continually declined. She maintained this state of mind as everything changed and challenged her, even when she could no longer walk, bathe, feed herself, or even move in bed.

So, after the pain became a persistent presence in my life, that favorite phrase of my mother's took on new meaning for me. And when the pain reared up again and again, I would take a calming breath and reassure myself, *This too shall pass*.

Appreciating the Valley

My acupuncturist, Pam, once explained to me that life does not go in a straight line and that there would be peaks and valleys. She said everyone thinks the high part of the cycle is normal and where we should be all the time. But with the high comes the low, and it is during these low times that we really grow and learn.

As time went on, I started to view the tough times not only as something to fear and endure but also as something to experience and learn from. Even though I couldn't wait for the pain to end, I began to appreciate the valley as a valuable growth catalyst.

One afternoon, I entered the elevator outside of Dr. Ryan's office. A woman in her seventies was standing in the corner of the elevator, and I couldn't help but notice the pain broadcasting from her stance and her eyes.

"You are really hurting today," I said with compassion.

"How do you know?" she replied.

I told her I had been there before and even felt despair. She confided she had horrible back pain but needed to get some medical issues under control before she could have surgery. The night before, she had felt deep despair.

I told her that, for me, the feeling of despair came in waves, but I always found something from within or without that kept me moving forward and out of the depths. She said that had been her experience, too. Then, we smiled at each other as we left the building.

Another woman who had overheard our conversation walked with me toward our cars. As we stood in the street facing each other, she said, "My friends wonder why I can be so positive after all the hard things I've had to endure. But it was those times that helped me grow and made me who I am today."

I replied, "This just popped into my head: The valley gives you depth!"

Relinquishing Control

I always thought that it was my duty to have a quality life and I could control what happened to me if I just worked hard enough. Consequently, at the very beginning of my pain, I felt like I had done something wrong. Once, I even told Alex, "I'm really sorry. It is like you had your choice of trains at the station, and you picked the wrong one—the one that broke down."

However, after a year of living with the illness, my journal reflected a change in perspective:

> *Now, I realize that I need to experience my life, not achieve it! I can't control everything. I have to let my life flow and do my best within the highs and lows.*

Two years into the pain, I told my acupuncturist, Pam, that my fears were starting to evaporate, including my fears of death, confrontation, not achieving, and not being loved.

In response, she said, "Life is really a journey of spiritual growth. When you are aware of your inner strength, you don't need to control what happens in your life as much and you have less fear."

Traveling with New Eyes

My journal at sixteen months into the illness shows how the painful load had shifted my perceptions of both my external and internal worlds:

> *Jackie told me today that she felt bad for me because my world had gotten so small. She's right. I no longer work, volunteer, or do social things. Sometimes, just trying to get out of pain consumes my whole day, and I feel sidelined from life. I hate these days. Somehow, I know that peace means accepting them. But what I didn't tell her was that as these external boundaries have gotten smaller, my internal world has completely opened up.*

When I was more in touch with my inner self, my view of the world started to shift. This change is described in this journal entry written two years into the pain:

> *When Alex and I were enduring a time-share presentation in Hawaii, the salesperson asked what I wanted to experience and see before I died—what was on my bucket list. I told her that I honestly did not have a bucket list and was content to go wherever life took me. She probably*

thought I was just trying to get out of the sale! But really, I've learned that I don't need to travel far to see beauty and to have rich experiences. When your heart is open, you can see the world in your own backyard.

About this time, my husband's company newsletter came in the mail, and this quote by Marcel Proust clearly summarized my experience:

"The voyage of discovery is not in seeking new landscapes but in having new eyes."

Picturing Spiritual Reconnection

Several times during the first year of pain, I woke up with a crystal clear image in my mind, which I then described in my journal.

The first time this happened was three months into my pain:

I am walking down a long, curving path. The trees are arching over, and it is so dark. The pain is like a huge pack on my back. Sometimes, Alex walks beside me. He can't carry the pack, but he waits with me when I rest.

Then, six months into my pain, the image reappeared:

I am still walking on that path, but now there is sunlight outlining the canopy of leaves overhead. I can see a round, brilliant, yellow sun up in the sky at the end of the trail.

Nine months into my pain, the mental picture made another morning appearance:

I'm still walking on that curved path, but today the sunlight overhead fills my chest. Sometimes, the trees arch over and it gets dark, but then this inner light guides me down the trail.

These images were comforting to me because they clearly depicted the spiritual growth I was experiencing at the time. During my first year of pain, I realized there was more to life than I had previously known and somehow I was personally connected to all of it. This knowledge moved from a pleasant thought in my mind to a resounding feeling deep within.

Two years into my pain, I was looking through our family photos and gasped when I saw a picture of me taken by my husband thirteen years before when we were hiking on the Oregon coast. In the picture, I am walking alone down a curving path with the sunlight peeking through the canopy of leaves over my head. It is the exact image that repeatedly popped into my mind during that first year of pain.

At that point in my journey, the coincidence of this old picture matching my repeated morning images shouldn't have surprised me, because over the years, information that helped point the way forward had kept coming in from old and new sources.

This chapter contains just a few ways in which I received meaningful information—such as images in my mind, pictures from my past, writings in an old journal, select memories, random comments from strangers, and timely quotes—that inspired me. These messages were often provocative, validating, and encouraging, and they seemed to push me down the healing path.

7

Recognizing the Body-Mind-Spirit Connection

During my first two years of pain, I started to suspect that my discomfort was more than just a breakdown of my body and that all parts of me (body, mind, and spirit) were linked and contributing in some way to my painful condition. My caregivers hinted at these ideas from the very beginning of my illness, but the concepts became real for me only through my direct personal experiences. Through this process, I gradually adopted a more holistic view of my condition.

The Emotional Theory

At the very beginning of my illness, each of my caregivers, one by one, gently brought up the possible link between my emotions and my pain. At the time, I was so focused on my physical pain that the idea that there may be an emotional component to my illness didn't sink in. I listened just long enough to record the ideas in my journal.

During my first appointment with Dr. Chalfin, he told me there was a strong connection between the bladder and the lower levels of the brain that participated in the processing of emotions (the limbic system).

The following week Dr. Ryan told me, "Interstitial cystitis is often a disease of misplaced emotions."

At my first psychotherapy session with Jackie, she said that her bladder pain had begun right after her brother died. He was driving drunk when he was killed, so along with the sadness, she'd felt a lot of anger. She'd even told her doctor that she thought her bladder was just really pissed off!

About five months into the pain during a visit with Dr. Ryan, I told her my bladder had been hurting a lot more over the past few weeks, and when the pain decreased a bit, I could tell that my whole nervous system was ramped up and in overdrive. She thought I would get better once I had worked awhile with Jackie on the emotional level. She told me that people can internalize issues for only so long before the body starts telling them it is breaking down. "You may be able to fix things mentally," Dr. Ryan encouraged, "But healing emotionally and physically takes time."

When I began my acupuncture sessions with Pam, she explained that the whole pelvic area and the bladder, in particular, were shaped like a vessel. She told me people often hold emotions, especially negative ones, in this part of the body.

Over time, each of my primary caregivers suggested a possible connection between my pain and my emotions.

Getting Testy About the Emotional Theory

Although learning about the effect emotions can have on pain was helpful, I bristled a bit whenever a caregiver brought up the subject. My body was really hurting, and I definitely didn't want my physical illness to be dismissed as being based solely on emotions!

This frustration is apparent in my journal entry nine months into my pain:

> *I think Dr. Noblett considers my pain to be almost completely related to my emotions. I feel judged when she says this, as if it is all in my control and if I continue to do poorly, it is because I couldn't get my act together. It is more complicated than this, and there are other pieces to my pain.*

> *Julie says the mind-body connection is very strong in me and that I have suffered through lots of emotional trauma. I don't think this is true; I have had the same types of emotional bumps and bruises as the average person. The mind-body connection is probably a factor in everyone; I am just willing to look at these issues in myself. There is a physical component to this illness, too. There may be a relationship between my emotions and*

the pain, but that doesn't mean the pain can be explained away solely as a byproduct of my feelings.

Jackie said that the emotional aspect was just one piece of the puzzle, and it was natural to be angry when I felt a caregiver was blaming all my physical issues on emotional triggers. She said that taking in all these different viewpoints about my condition was important, but it was up to me to decide what information fit me.

Toward the end of the first year, I made some peace with the concept that my emotions were related to my pain level as evidenced by my journal entry from this time:

I have a true physical illness: My bladder is red and inflamed, and my pelvic-floor muscles are in knots. But my pain is being transmitted by the nervous system, which has lots of pathways that are all connected and influence each other. So there are many different neural connections that can influence my perception of the pain and how bad or how good I feel. In short, even though the pain is not all in my head, what is happening in my head can really influence my pain.

Experiencing the Mind–Body Link

Over the years, many experiences helped me come to appreciate the link between my emotional state and my pelvic pain. In the early days of the illness, I noticed that any time Alex was out of town on business, I could count on a flare-up of my bladder pain. Likewise, in stressful situations, like sitting in on a time-share presentation or returning a lamp to a very rude salesperson, I would actually feel my pelvic-floor muscles tighten up.

I also noticed that positive emotions, too, had an effect on my body. For example, calming experiences, like walking at night, attending yoga class, and hugging Alex, could make my pelvic pain drop.

Another experience of the mind-body connection happened in reverse: Working on my body could bring about an emotional release. For example, about eighteen months into the pain, I began a yoga class that combined meditation with long-held postures aimed at stretching out the hip and pelvic areas. While I was quietly enduring a prolonged stretch for my hips (pigeon pose), tears just started pouring out, wetting my face and the mat below me. This was really strange because there was nothing upsetting me at the moment that would warrant such an outburst. But when the crying stopped, I felt so much better.

I quietly used my socks to wipe my runny nose and tried to slink out of the studio. Several of my classmates stopped me and told me they'd had a similar experience. The instructor handed me a tissue, squeezed my arm, and asked if I were okay. (She probably saw me using my socks.) She told me that people often hold a lot of emotion in the areas around the pelvis and hips, and when those areas are opened up, it is common to have an emotional release.

My physical therapist, Julie, told me that quite a few of her patients experienced an emotional release when she worked on their bodies. I'd heard about this connection between the body and emotions in a few physical therapy classes when I was a student, but at the time I hadn't given it much merit. However, after I had personally experienced an emotional release while doing body-work on several occasions, the notion seemed more credible to me.

Nervous System Connections

Julie told me that pain doesn't always signal more damage to your body or a progression of the disease. Sometimes, the body's neurological system remembers and reproduces the pain even when there is no physical reason for it. When you have chronic pain, the pathways can fire on their own without any input from the originating sources of pain. The pain can result from these neural pathways being activated at the brain level, and many things, including emotions, can trigger them.

One instance of this happening stands out in my memory: Two years into my illness, my bladder pain flared up but then subsided within days, so it obviously wasn't a sign of ongoing inflammation or an organ in distress. Then, later that week while Alex and I were having a heated discussion, my bladder pain suddenly surfaced. There it was: Pain in response to turbulent emotion! When the argument passed, so did the bladder pain.

Alex questioned, "Why do you care whether it is coming from your brain or your bladder? Pain is pain."

He had a good point. But the source of the pain was important to me because when I knew where the pain was coming from, I knew which methods to use to get out of it. If there was a physical reason for the pain, such as severe inflammation or erosion of the bladder lining, then physical measures needed to be taken. On the other hand, if the pain was related to nervous-system pathways in overdrive, I needed to look for possible triggers for those pain pathways, which might be physical, psychosocial, emotional, or spiritual.

The good news was that the pain didn't necessarily signal more damage to my body. The bad news was that the areas of my nervous system that transmitted pain were now sensitized and easily activated. They could reproduce the pain on their own even when the area of my body that originally caused the pain was healed. I had to try to figure out how to calm them down. To give me hope, I would remind myself of something I knew from teaching in the neurological area: The brain is not a static entity, and its structure can change with practice and experience. Therefore, if I reinforced new pathways that were calming and pain-free, the over-sensitive pain pathways may eventually quiet down.

My Body, My Teacher

At first, pain was my enemy, and I would try anything and everything to get rid of it. But the longer the pain was part of my life, the more I realized that my discomfort was teaching me things. The pelvic pain would rear up when I felt stressed or unsafe, and this gave me clues about the inner issues I was carrying. My body's wisdom was no longer a whisper. It would shout my inner truth! For example, at a potluck with my girlfriends, I was sharing other people's business and letting out information that could have potentially hurt the ones I love. That night, I couldn't sleep and my rear end was in spasm. I swear, my body doesn't let me get away with anything anymore!

Over time, I was able to link more than just the pelvic pain to my emotions. When different parts of my body would become painful, there was often a connection between what I was feeling in my body and what I was feeling emotionally. For example, once when I was arguing with my husband, my heart started to hurt. The same pain—specifically, a spot between the fourth and fifth ribs on the left side of my sternum—would throb and feel tender to the touch when Alex and I were at odds with one another. One day, the pain began when he entered the room and quieted when he exited. When I described the heart pain to Dr. Ryan, she didn't even examine me. She just said the discomfort around my heart was related to the issues I was working through with my husband.

I suspect my body has always sent those messages, but I just wasn't tuned into them. In fact, my body had to scream in pain for years before I started to listen!

My pain became more than simply a reflection of physical disease; it evolved into an internal alert mechanism. The discomfort or feelings in my body signaled me when areas of my life or my person needed attention. My acupuncturist, Pam, told me that my pelvic pain had become my messenger and would let me know when I needed to get back to my center.

On one particularly discouraging day about two and a half years into my pain, Iben, my life coach, asked me if it might be possible to switch my perspective from being mad at my body for being in pain to having gratitude that it was trying to tell me something. In that moment, my response was a resounding "No!" Once in a while, though, I saw my pain less as an adversary pulling me out of my life and more as a friend signaling me to get the most out of my life.

However, not all physical complaints can be explained away as simply a spiritual and/or emotional message. We have a body, a biological system, and even the most spiritually advanced and emotionally healthy people get sick and die.

Today, I see physical symptoms as arising not totally from the body nor totally from the mind and/or spirit but as an indication that something is happening at all levels of my being. As Dr. Noblett told me: "We are mind, body, and spirit all together; they can't be separated."

Subconscious Releasing

About a year and a half into my pain, my body started to react spontaneously in many different ways. At first I wondered if these happenings were simply a sign that something else was going wrong with my body, but over time I began to appreciate that these subconscious activities were a part of my healing process. These direct experiences of subconscious releasing would continue and develop over the years to come.

Unwinding

Eighteen months into my illness, my physical therapist, Julie, noticed that my lower spine was very tight. She treated the area, and then told me to ask Pam if she could also address the problem with acupuncture.

So, during my next acupuncture session, Pam put needles in my left hand in a pattern that was related to spinal opening. After lying there for about fifteen minutes, I felt tingling in my left foot, which then progressed up my left leg. Slowly and spontaneously, my chin started to tuck and my neck elongated. It felt like my head was being gently pulled away from my body. I wasn't moving this way consciously; it was just happening to me. I could stop the movement at any time, but if I relaxed, it continued. It is an understatement to say that this was a really strange experience, but I wasn't afraid and didn't resist. The movement felt just like the cervical traction I had undergone to alleviate the pain of previous neck injuries, and that familiarity was comforting to me. It was also easier for me to accept because it was happening in response to Pam's treatment, and I knew that acupuncture had been healing for me in the past.

A few months later, I woke up one morning and my neck began moving just like it had during the acupuncture session. Then, every day for a full month, right when I woke up or right before I fell asleep, my body would spontaneously move as it had during acupuncture, with new movements being added to the repertoire. It started with neck movements in a forward or backward direction, followed by movements from side to side, and then rotation, and then combined motions of the neck. Next, my thorax started to move along with my neck, and then my lower back joined in, followed by my legs.

Soon after that, all areas of my body would activate and move in random ways. The pattern of muscle activation and the timing were always different. Sometimes, there would be long-held postures; other times, slow or fast oscillations would occur. At first, the movements happened only when I was relaxed in bed. But after a while, my entire body would move spontaneously whenever I allowed it and in any position, even standing.

I told Alex, "These movements are either a form of healing or a sign of pathology."

I knew there were many motor pathways below the conscious (cortical) levels of the brain, but I had only seen them activated in my patients who'd had injuries to the nervous system. The pathological movements I had seen in my patients were usually in a typical movement pattern and not easily stopped once activated, and they often interfered with the patient's functioning. I was relieved that my movements were varied and random, that I could stop them at any time, and that they never interfered with function. If the movements were happening with my legs or trunk, I was always fully aware and could simultaneously talk or perform complicated activities with my arms and hands.

During this time, my friend Lisa came over for lunch one day. As physical therapists, we both had spent a lot of time analyzing movement. So I lay on the couch and said, "Watch this." Then, I let my body do its thing.

Lisa's eyes got really wide, and she took two steps backward.

"I know; it's weird," I said. "Thank goodness I wasn't born in the past, when I could have been burned at the stake for this type of thing!"

I asked Lisa to compare the movement when I just let it happen with when I tried to reproduce it volitionally. She said the first movement looked much more fluid and coordinated.

When I showed the movements to each of my doctors, they said they had never seen motions like that before. They told me it was obvious the movements were not in my conscious control, but they didn't think they were pathological. Both Dr. Ryan and Dr. Noblett hypothesized that it might be a way my body was releasing energy and trying to heal itself.

My physical therapist, Julie, said my movements looked like those she had seen others perform during a Myofascial Release course she had taken. In this course, these movements were called "unwinding."

Although my movements were often random, my pelvis often rotated to the left and my neck often turned to the right. Stella and Pam described my movements from the yoga perspective as a kundalini-type movement. Later, Iben gave the counterclockwise rotation the nickname "the vortex" and explained it as a way my body was releasing energy and trying to ground itself.

These theories seemed to match my physical experiences. The movement seemed to be related to moving or releasing energy, because once the movement stopped, I would feel light tingling throughout my body, similar to how I felt during other energy work, like acupuncture and Reiki. The movements also seemed to be related to a release of tension in the muscles and tissues of my body.

One time when Julie was working internally trying to manually release a pelvic-floor muscle spasm, my spine went into its spontaneous movement. As I moved, she noticed that the tough, fibrous band of tissue that she was working on completely softened and felt like normal tissue.

I think the movements were related to healing, because my overall discomfort lessened as soon as these movements began and because, when I was in pain and would let the movements happen, my pain level would drop. Even the idea that the movements contributed to grounding me didn't seem far off, because I noticed that after the movements, sometimes my arches would be lower and I'd get a more solid, weight-bearing sensation through my feet.

Facial Movements

The next thing I noticed was that sometimes my eyes would spontaneously shut tight and the muscles of my forehead would contract, deepening the creases between my eyes. Once these muscles were activated, I could easily relax my face. The first time it happened, I was stretching out my hips and pelvic area during a long-held yoga pose (pigeon pose).

Soon, this facial reaction began to occur whenever I was experiencing some strong emotion or working through some tough issue with Iben. She said it looked like the face of a child saying, "No, I don't want to see that!" She was right. The facial movement seemed to happen when the situation was emotionally charged for me. It was almost as if I were trying to slow down or shut off my insight into something difficult or painful.

Gone were the days when I could hide my emotions. Now, my face would give me a clue that I was feeling something. When the squinting happened spontaneously, I knew I was uncovering an issue and it would reveal itself in time.

As I worked through the layers and healed, this reaction happened less and less. Now, it shows up on rare occasions when I am experiencing or uncovering some deeply held emotion.

Dreaming

Most of my acupuncture sessions began with Pam asking about my dreaming. The first time she asked, though, I was surprised and wondered aloud how she knew I was having unusual dreams. Then, I told her about my movie-like, Technicolor dreams with convoluted plots that seemed to go on for hours.

Pam explained that my pulses showed heat in the heart, which could be related to spiritual or emotional churning, and that my description of vivid, full-color dreams was right out of her acupuncture textbook under "heat in the heart." This energy could then travel to the bladder and cause the pain to flare up.

Some of these dreams were so clear in their imagery that they needed absolutely no interpretation. On a few occasions, I even woke up with the knowledge that I had worked through something significant.

Exhalation and Excretion

Two and a half years into my pain, I began working with Iben, a practitioner who combined multi-dimensional life coaching with energetic bodywork. After my second treatment, my body began spontaneously exhaling, sometimes with a vocal tone attached and sometimes without any vocalization. The exhalation was more prolonged than any deep breathing I'd done before, and it felt different than simply letting out air after a big breath. After about ten minutes, my breathing pattern would normalize, and I would feel more peaceful.

After each of the first few sessions with Iben, I also had diarrhea for two days afterward, even though I didn't feel sick. Iben reassured me that this was common and a good sign I was releasing inner blockages and toxins. I had no idea what was going on, but deep down I had a gut feeling that it was healing.

I told Dr. Ryan about the diarrhea, exhalation, and dreaming.

Looking at me with amazement and happiness, she said, "This experience has been so good for you. Very few people are open enough to experience this type of healing because they don't want to look at what they are carrying. When you are little and things happen, you close things up to keep surviving. But sooner or later, it has to come out."

Embracing the Body-Mind-Spirit Connection

One evening during a rain shower, another woman and I ran side-by-side from our cars into the grocery store. Once inside, we both laughed about the surprising downpour. I'm not sure how we got started, but we ended up standing in front of the produce section talking about our pain and the connections between the mind and body that each of us had experienced.

Kristi had suffered for years with major back pain and fibromyalgia. She shared with me how, through hypnosis and psychotherapy, she had learned to go into a meditative state to relieve her pain and no longer needed medications.

Surprisingly, Kristi's daughter suffered from interstitial cystitis, just like me. While we were talking, it dawned on her that her daughter's pelvic pain might have some link to the abduction and sexual abuse she had suffered at age nine.

Kristi mentioned that she wanted to share her personal experiences with the mind-body connection, but she did not think people would take her seriously because she had a history of bipolar disorder and alcohol abuse, and at one point in her illness, she had become addicted to prescription painkillers. I knew that her experiences of the mind-body connection could be true because I had directly experienced the power of this connection myself. Kristi told me she was happy I was writing about my experience because I had a credible voice. Of course, this so-called credibility may totally depend upon the perception of the reader.

I told my husband, Alex, that I had started this book as my professional self and ended up talking about things quite out of mainstream experience. Honestly, sometimes I hear myself telling a friend a story and just shake my head at how crazy this would have sounded to me just a few short years ago. My rational, scientific mind would have discounted many of these experiences, and I probably would have rolled my eyes and shut the book. But as I worked to get out of pain, things kept happening to me, and over time, I just accepted these experiences as part of my healing path. My direct experiences shifted my perception, and my past skepticism gradually transformed into openness and awe.

Realizing that my body wasn't just causing problems for me gave me some comfort. On some level, my body seemed to have its own intelligence. It seemed to be trying to heal itself and was giving me messages about other parts of me that needed healing, too.

Over the first two years of pain, I gradually became aware of a connection between my physical pain and my emotional state. At that point in my recovery, I had no idea how much more I would learn about this connection and that working on my emotional/spiritual issues would be the major way I would eventually heal my body.

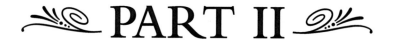

PART II

Healing Through the Layers

"Deep unspeakable suffering may well be called a baptism, a regeneration, the initiation into a new state."
— George Eliot

8

Mining the Depths

After working for two years to decrease my pain and cure my physical condition, my pain had dropped from persistent to occasional and from debilitating to annoying. Since I had exhausted many of the options for physical treatment, my focus now turned progressively inward in an effort to uncover the emotional/spiritual issues that were contributing to a ramp-up of my nervous system and the continuation of my physical pain. I started this introspection because I thought it might be a way to become pain-free. I had no idea this process would help heal my mind and spirit, too.

A New Path

Two years into my illness, I was feeling good both mentally and physically, and most of my days were pain-free. I was doing so well that Jackie discharged me from psychotherapy and Julie discharged me from physical therapy, and I only needed to attend massage therapy and acupuncture once a month to manage my condition.

Then, in early October of 2009, after six months of being dormant, the bladder pain came back. This time, the pain level was in the mild range (three on a scale of one to ten), and it bothered me for ten to thirty percent of the day. By then, I'd spent eighteen months in physical therapy and psychotherapy, attended eighty acupuncture sessions, and endured numerous bladder instillations and trigger-point injections. Although I was grateful that my pain level was no longer debilitating, I was also really discouraged that it kept coming back, especially after I had worked so hard to heal.

My journal from this time clearly depicts my disappointment:

I'm mad about having to be sick, and I'm mad at my body. I want to be normal. I don't want this pelvic pain. I don't want it to be such a part of my life. Today I feel like damaged goods; I feel sorry for myself.

I began attending acupuncture on a weekly basis to help manage the discomfort. When I wasn't improving after several treatments, Pam suggested I make an appointment with Iben Larssen, a new practitioner in her office. Pam explained that Iben had traveled the globe for over twenty years gathering skills in a multitude of alternative healing methods.

When Pam initially suggested I work with Iben, I thought she might be pushing me off on someone else because she didn't know how to help me anymore. Pam picked up on my skepticism without me saying a word. She told me that sometimes she had an intuitive sense about the direction her patients should go in order to heal, and she had a gut feeling that working with Iben would help me.

Pam explained that people can hold experiences within their bodies that can cause physical pain. She said that going deeper to uncover these old beliefs and life patterns was similar to mining. While I had a flashlight to guide my work, Iben had a bright headlamp and her insight could help me figure out where to dig.

Like most of the population, I wasn't clamoring for an opportunity to work with an emotional or spiritual advisor. I had already learned so much from my illness and had recently graduated from psychotherapy with a gold star of self-awareness. What could possibly have accumulated in just a few months off the therapy couch? I didn't think I had much else to uncover.

I was wrong.

Starting in November of 2009, Iben and I worked together consistently for a year and sporadically, as needed, since then, up to the present day. Iben combines energetic bodywork with multi-dimensional life coaching. During each session, we spend time talking, and Iben gives me topics on which to do introspective work in between our visits. Afterward, she places her hands lightly in different locations on my clothed, reclining body. I almost always feel a light tingling throughout my body and relaxation creeping over me.

Especially in the beginning, Iben encouraged me to look into the deeper parts of me, and gradually subconscious patterns in my thinking and life came clearly into view. Sometimes, I would become aware of painful dynamics in my life and my contribution to the way things were. At times, I would get mad at her and think, *Why the hell did you turn on the lights!* But once those lights were on, there was no going back. The process was difficult and painful at times, but never frightening. What I was uncovering I already knew at some level, so it was never foreign. It was my truth. And I had a friend with me on the journey. Iben created a space of love and compassion, and she walked next to me, all the while prodding me down the path deeper into myself.

Deciding to Share

The first draft of this book didn't include any of the information in this chapter. Since we each have our own emotional issues, I initially thought that sharing mine would limit the scope of the book and make it less useful to others. I also thought that if what I'd learned through my deeper introspection departed from the perspective of the readers, they might discount other parts of the book that might be helpful for them. Finally, this information is very personal, and I wasn't really sure I wanted to expose myself that much.

But the benefits of sharing kept coming up, and eventually they outweighed my previous concerns. First, Julie, Iben, and Chris told me that their other clients with pelvic pain shared many of my internal struggles. Second, when I shared Iben's insights with others, I noticed that some of what she said lit up with meaning for other people, too. They would often be very grateful for the different perspective that Iben's simple words offered. Third, Iben explained that through developing this book, I had transitioned from patient to teacher, and in that role, sharing personal experiences was often helpful to others. That made sense to me because almost every one of my caregivers had generously and openly shared stories from their lives when it could help me. Finally, after my cousin

Rich, who is a professional writer, read my first draft, he questioned me about parts that were incomplete or didn't ring true. I had to laugh because all the information that would fill in the gaps was in my journal, written during my time with Iben. I just hadn't let the reader in far enough.

The biggest reason I couldn't leave out this section, though, is because this introspection has been crucial to my recovery, and during that process, my pelvic pain completely quieted down. My bladder pain actually stopped and did not return for a full year.

My healing went beyond my physical body, too. Once I really looked at and processed what I was carrying deep inside, the issues and hurts I had ruminated over throughout my life no longer had a hold on my heart and mind. They were still a part of me, but I saw them from a higher vantage point, and because I wasn't enmeshed in those life patterns, they no longer defined me. No longer encumbered by this past stuff, I felt so free. I landed more firmly into my authentic self, and my life began to transform.

My experience is but one example of the self-discovery process and the healing potential of looking within. I realize that some of my experiences may not resonate with others or be in line with their particular life views. I totally understand this disparity, because before this illness, parts of my story would have sounded simply outrageous to me and I would have wondered about the sanity of the writer. So I am not offended if you don't make it to the end. I know that some of my personal discovery will land in the lap of those for whom it is meant, and that is the reason I've written this book. With that said, get ready to jump into the deep end!

Choosing the Journey

While I sipped tea in the comfortable waiting area, Iben walked toward me with a slight spring in her step and a clipboard poised at her midsection.

During our first hour together, Iben listened as I told her a little about my mother, my traumatic birth, and mostly, my experiences with pelvic pain. Then, I reclined on her treatment table, and she put her hands gently on my fully clothed body. I didn't feel anything until she placed her hands over my lower pelvic region, at which point I felt a vibration under her hands, like Reiki on steroids.

"It's all stuck here," she said.

After the examination, I sat up and Iben told me her impressions. Here are the main points of her analysis, as I wrote in my journal that night:

- *My spirit did not fully enter my body at birth. In other words, I did not fully incarnate. I often lived my life through others, and I hadn't fully experienced my own body and my own life.*
- *When I told her of my increased insight and peace, she said I'd had a glimpse of being centered but hadn't fully landed yet.*
- *In the past, I didn't love without expectation, and that's why it didn't always flow back. Accompanying this loving energy were neediness and fear of abandonment, and these thoughts and emotions helped create negative relationships and experiences in my life.*
- *Intense resentment that is not expressed often goes to the bladder (literally, being pissed off). In our society, women suffer from interstitial cystitis more often than men because we are not given permission to show anger, so we hold it within our bodies.*
- *I have an open "third eye." I am very intuitive, but this was never supported by my mother during my childhood and by the people who surrounded me throughout my life.*
- *I am mostly yin (female) energy, and my mom was mostly yang (male) energy.*
- *When I showed Iben my spontaneous body movements, she said my body was moving to become grounded and was turning me to the left, the feminine side.*
- *I have a low libido (which was no surprise to me!).*
- *"When you are aligned with who you think you should be rather than with whom you truly are, the body will try to call you back to center."*

Almost everything Iben said seemed strange and disturbing. The concepts and language were totally different than how I had been taught to view the world. I wondered what I had gotten myself into. I told a few people at the gym about her impressions, and we all agreed it was crazy stuff.

But along with all that resistance, I had a gut feeling that some of what she said was true and I needed to travel this path. What is more, my pain levels dropped after the first session with Iben, which made me even more interested in returning for more treatment. But my husband, Alex, was against it. He said I was in pain and vulnerable and that Iben was no better than a snake-oil salesman. For two weeks I agonized, torn by a desire to return and a fear of being taken advantage of.

My journal describes this internal conflict:

> I went to see Iben for one session and I want to go back, but Alex is stopping me, and this is creating a conflict for me. I don't want to make him mad, because he is my main support and I need him. Anything good for me would not tear us apart. I am drawn to Iben and want to work with her, but Alex is dead set against it and thinks I'm getting ripped off. I'm mad at him for directing my journey, but then he only has my best interests at heart. I am vulnerable now, and it has spun me up and increased my anxiety, which isn't good for my pain. I need to accept my relationships, my loneliness, and my illness. But I don't want to!

Looking back, this was a turning point for me. I had to choose whether I wanted to embark on this new path in my life, knowing that saying yes to this process meant challenging my husband's resistance. Part of me was saying, *Suck it up and maintain the status quo*, and another part of me was saying, *It's time to look at your pain, yourself, and your life.*

Finally, I talked about my dilemma with Pam (my acupuncturist) and Julie (my physical therapist). They both told me about other patients with my condition who'd had really positive results from their work with Iben. Even Dr. Ryan chimed in with encouragement. She explained that Alex was an engineer and thought in more concrete ways, so the type of work Iben did would be hard for him to accept. She said the treatment was worth trying because I'd had good results with Reiki and, especially, because Iben was someone Pam trusted.

Before my illness, I never would have been open to working with Iben, but my experiences over the first two painful years had left my mind a bit more open. I couldn't deny that yoga and meditation helped decrease my pain, and I knew I didn't need to become a yogi or a Buddhist in order to reap some of the benefits of these ancient healing traditions. I knew I didn't have to fully agree with Iben or adopt her belief system to give the process a chance. So I decided to continue the work with Iben and let my body determine whether this path was healing for me.

Grounding

After my first session, Iben gave me homework. I was to sit in a chair with my feet flat on the floor and breathe deeply for five minutes each morning and evening. She also asked me to write about my life from the perspective of my soul, including why my soul would have chosen these relationships and these life experiences.

When I decided to return for more sessions with Iben, I sat down and wrote the story of my birth.

Six weeks before my anticipated birth date, my mother started hemorrhaging while doing the dishes. She yelled to my dad to get some towels, and they sped to the hospital, where I arrived in an emergent rush. My mother required two blood transfusions and barely survived. When I reached adulthood, she confided that during my birth she'd seen the proverbial white light at the end of a long tunnel and had a sense of incredible peace. She remembered thinking, *If this is dying, it's not that bad.* But she didn't go into the light and eventually went home to recuperate without me.

I spent the first six weeks of my life in the hospital. My weight dropped from five pounds at birth to three pounds, and one night they called my parents to let them know I probably wouldn't make it until morning. Father John, a Catholic priest and very close friend, drove over to bless me in the hospital. My mother, a devout Catholic, changed my name from Ruth Marie to Mary Ruth and dedicated me to Mary, the mother of Jesus.

I started our second session by reading my birth story to Iben. Afterward, she repeated one of her first impressions: that it probably had been difficult for my soul to come fully into my body because I subconsciously knew that being born would endanger my mother. She also suggested that because of this early trauma, part of me might have felt like a burden, abandoned, and alone.

Iben also explained that my name, Mary, is the female (yin) form of Christ's loving energy and that the name Marie meant love and compassion. I had never liked my name, but now I embraced it.

Lying there on the table in Iben's treatment room, it felt oddly like being christened all over again. Iben gave significance to my name and welcomed me into the world.

As I was driving home from this second appointment, I started to exhale spontaneously, and the air resonated with a deep tone. My abdominal muscles contracted, and my pelvis rotated to the left. Then, I felt my intestines cramping, and I made it home just in time for a dumping incident. Alex took over the dinner duties. While I was lying on the couch feeling really wiped out, a light tingling started in my midsection, traveled down both legs, and then concentrated in my left leg.

The whole next week, my emotions were heightened. I was touched by acts of kindness all around me, and tears frequently rolled down my cheeks. All week, my bladder was pain-free, my pelvic-floor muscles were more relaxed, and I had increased energy. On two occasions, my eyes squinted shut and I felt a crinkling sensation at the base of my brain. This happened when Alex was intense and negative with our son and when he touched me in a sexual way.

As I walked up the stairs to the treatment room for my third session, I saw Iben standing at the top of the stairs scanning my body. I remembered that during our first appointment, she'd told me she had always been able to see the energy field, or aura, that surrounded people. I laughed and said, "So how do I look?" She replied, "Last week your aura was scattered and above you, but today it is more compact and it goes all the way down to your toes."

When we were in the treatment room, I told her about the diarrhea and dumping I'd experienced after my last session. She said many people experience diarrhea after the first sessions as toxins are released, and that, counter-intuitively, this was a good sign.

When I told her about my eyes closing and feeling a crinkling sensation in my brain, Iben said shutting my eyes tight was probably related to my resistance to feeling the emotions and humanness of my life now that I was more present. She also mentioned that the area between the eyes is correlated with spiritual insight (the third eye) and that contracting my brow might be slowing down the flow of information. She told me to not worry about these reactions; they would subside over time.

She was right about my resistance to feeling my emotions. I wanted to gloss over this process instead of going through it. I kept telling myself, *It's better now. I'm fine; I'm fine; I'm fine.* But I wasn't fine, and I had to go through it.

Is It Right?

In the beginning, I often wondered whether it was right to go through this process—a hesitation I knew was grounded in my past. My mother definitely would have considered this prolonged introspection to be self-indulgent and egotistical. She often told me I had a very active mind and should keep it busy, because it would take me places I didn't want to go. So I'd always had a fear of what I would uncover in quiet solitude.

When I told Iben about this hesitation, she suggested, "Instead of asking whether something is right or wrong, ask if it is life-giving." She said that when you ask if something is right or wrong, you tap into your mind and belief system, producing a value judgment. In contrast, when you ask if it's life-giving, you tap into your soul. She said that you often choose a course of action because it is life-giving for yourself, and occasionally, you sacrifice because it is life-giving for your family or community.

Iben reassured me that looking at deeper issues wasn't self-centered or egotistical. Then, she said, "The term 'egoism' comes from Latin and simply means 'being me.'"

Over time, I realized that going through this process was life-giving not only for me but also for others around me, including my children.

Several years after I began working with Iben, when my daughter was going through a difficult time, I encouraged her by saying that suffering is really an opportunity to grow. She said she knew that was true because she'd watched me evolve as I went through my illness. She told me I'd changed a lot and was very open now and that she also felt she could confide in me.

My son, who is now an older teenager, told me recently that he'd had a difficult time as a child in our home. He confided that he always knew I loved him, but I was so wrapped up in getting validation that I wasn't there for him emotionally. He often felt unseen and unsupported in our family.

He said that when I healed emotionally during my illness, I changed and the dynamics in our home changed, and as a result, his life got much better.

Revisiting Relationships

When I look back on my journey with Iben, it seems to have gone in cycles. I would go inward and uncover some truths, and then my focus would move outward, and I would see and experience my life in a new way. My internal work was often reflected in the changes in my life, and the challenges of my life would drive more internal work. So it makes sense that after this initial grounding work, I began to look out at my life.

During my first weeks of working with Iben, I told her about my daily experiences, often focusing on the times when my connection with others was strained or the love I expressed was not reflected back to me. During these interactions, I would often feel my pelvic floor tense up, so I knew they were stressful and related to my pain. Over time, I realized that I resented when people in my life did not meet my expectations for emotional connection or support. I remembered many of these infractions and kept them neatly cataloged in my mind. Almost every one of my caregivers linked pelvic and bladder pain with holding negative emotions, especially anger. So it seemed appropriate to look at my relationships with other people.

Iben used the following analogies and philosophies to help me see these interactions from a different perspective.

The Cross

I confided to Iben that I often felt isolated and lonely. She asked me to write the word "Alone" and then to add an "I"—changing "Alone" to "All One." She told me that in solitude you connect with the one power that is bigger than all of us—the energy that is all around us, resides in each of us, and connects us all.

Next, Iben had me draw a cross. She explained that the vertical line symbolized my connection with the All One (a.k.a. God) and the horizontal line symbolized my connection with other people. She said my connection to the All One was needed to support my connection with others.

Oceans and Paper Cups

Iben explained that not everyone is capable of giving at the level I gave and desired (or demanded) to be given in return. She told me I had a big capacity for deep, emotional connection. She said that if water were used as an analogy for this type of connection, I could hold a lot. I was like an ocean. She explained that not everyone had this ability, and some people were like paper cups.

This analogy clearly depicted many of my past experiences with people. Often, I flowed out this ocean of mine to connect with other people, and I just ended up swamping them, instead. And when I flowed out this ocean and only a paper cupful flowed back, I was often confused, hurt, and angry. I wondered why all these people were withholding their ocean and whether maybe I wasn't loveable enough to receive the full amount.

Iben explained that when someone gives me a paper cupful of connection, sometimes that is all they have, and in some cases, that cup is a huge sacrifice.

Mirrors

Iben often compared people to mirrors. She described people who inspire us as upright mirrors, people who repulse us as upside-down mirrors, and people who initially impress us but later repel us as smoky mirrors. She stated that all types of mirrors are valuable because they reflect back information about who we choose to be. She explained that I am a mirror for other people, too, and I may reflect to others their inability or resistance to go into deeper levels of self awareness. She warned that some people will turn away from me because they are uncomfortable with this insight.

Frequency and Filters

Iben said we are all tuned in to different frequencies of energy and information. She used the analogy of different radio stations, explaining that I may be tuned in to rock while another person may be tuned in to jazz. Because of this difference, our communication may not be optimal. She theorized that, eventually, the people who are tuned in to a different frequency than I am will move away from my life and those who are tuned in to the same frequency will come closer.

Iben explained that each of us also has a filter through which we process information and view the world, like a pair of prescription eyeglasses unique to that person. These filters are the product of our life experiences and can be influenced by gender, culture, religion, personal history, and traumatic experiences. New experiences, too, can alter our filters, which, in turn, can alter our perceptions. I have personally experienced this type of shift.

During my first month of intense pain, my friend Sandy gave me the memoir *Eat, Pray, Love: One Woman's Search for Everything Across Italy, India, and Indonesia*, by Elizabeth Gilbert, which had just been published and went on to become a best-seller and then a movie starring Julia Roberts. At the time, I thought the author was somewhat self-indulgent and had created her own problems (as depicted in the book). The only part that resonated with me at the time was when the author compared her bladder pain to being stabbed with a red-hot poker. If I were to read the book now, I would appreciate her journey at a much deeper level—because, over time, my experiences have changed what I'm tuned into, and now her message would easily permeate my filters.

In my relationships, I used to spend much of my time reading people's reactions and adjusting myself to meet their needs or to get their approval. Iben told me that it was not my responsibility to hide or change myself to match the frequency of another person or to try to permeate their filters. She encouraged me to not hide my strength and my self. My homework was to become more aware of when I put myself in either a superior or inferior role in order to be liked.

Responsibility

Iben told me I was responsible for my own actions and reactions, but I was not accountable for someone else's behavior. I had no control over it. To summarize, she said, "You are one hundred percent responsible for your fifty percent of the relationship."

She explained that when someone was reacting negatively toward me, I had several choices: I could leave it up to them to tell me what they needed; I could ask them to clarify what was going on; or I could assume what they were thinking. However, she said, the third option was just making movies in my head because I could never really know someone else's reality.

I am about a decade younger than my sister and two brothers, and I was often hurt and disappointed that we did not have a closer connection. During our occasional visits, my modus operandi was to rush in and spill my guts with a zeal that, if articulated in words, would have screamed, "Like me, like me, like me!"

A few days after Iben talked with me about my responsibility for my relationships with others, my sister and her husband came over for dinner. They live across the country from me, and it was the first time since the onset of my illness that I had seen them. At one point during the evening, I noticed my daughter, Katherine, standing in front of her wall of medals enthusiastically talking about her college plans. I thought my sister looked a bit intimidated. In the past, I would have rushed in to tone down Katherine's exuberance and to prop up my sister's ego. But this time I didn't try to control the reactions of my guests; I gave them space to just be. I focused mainly on what I was putting out there and what I was feeling inside. To my surprise, my pelvic floor was relaxed the whole night, and I didn't have any bladder pain. My guests responded with openness, kindness, and real sharing. On his way out the door, my brother-in-law hugged me and said it was our best visit ever.

Hierarchy

On my next session with Iben following my sister and brother-in-law's visit, I said, "You know, I have always lived in a hierarchy. It was everywhere in my life—at home, at school, in my community, and even in my church."

Although, at the time, I was just sharing a thought, it became clear over time that my reaction to hierarchy had always been intense, even when it wasn't outwardly expressed. For the first few years of my pain, nothing made my symptoms flare up more than feeling like I was being pushed into a subordinate role. When I put myself into this lower role by "shrinking to fit," I would often experience pelvic-floor tightness, bladder pain, or dumping. I suppose we all have issues that trigger us, and hierarchy was one of mine.

From as early as I can remember, I have always been keenly aware of hierarchies between people. That doesn't mean I was above it all, either. Throughout my life, I strove for validation from those in a "superior" position: my parents, my siblings, popular kids at school, teachers, bosses, and so on. I always wanted to be the favorite daughter or sister, the star student or employee. Although I also championed the underdog and acted kindly toward others, hierarchy often tainted even these actions. Part of my underlying motivation was to feel superior, to be better in the eyes of others, and perhaps even better in the eyes of God.

Hierarchy was also intertwined with my drive for achievement. I have a clear memory of standing in my brother's bedroom at age thirteen and thinking I would never be the prettiest or the most popular but I could be the smartest. From that point on, I drove myself academically.

Through working with Iben, I started to appreciate that beneath this need to achieve was an all-consuming desire to feel loved and connected. Whenever I felt a lack of connection with others, my internal drive for achievement became even greater. This energy pushed away people even more, thus creating a vicious cycle.

Iben explained that in a hierarchy, it is difficult to experience pure, unconditional love. She asked me to imagine looking at a city from a low vantage point, where I could see that everything had varying heights. Then, she had me imagine looking at the same city from high above; with this view, everything seemed to lie on a single plane. Iben explained that insight means seeing things from a higher vantage point, and this perception comes from a connection with God (the All One). I'd had occasional glimpses of this higher vision before, and over time I started adopting this view more and more in my life.

Intimacy

About this time, I wrote a memoir about the lessons I'd learned from my mother during her illness, which I was planning to send to my sister. Just as I was patting myself on the back for this kind and benevolent act, it dawned on me that my positive intentions were accompanied by negative ones. I wanted to receive love and respect from my sister for being wise and insightful, and I wanted to show her I had a bond with our mother that she didn't have. Yikes! I had never seen this dark side of myself before!

When I told my neighbors Kelly and Lee about this underlying motivation, instead of looking at me with disdain, they actually stepped closer.

Iben explained that sharing my negative side showed my humanness and allowed my friends to be human, too. "This is intimacy: Into me you see," she said.

I started to see that there was a hierarchy within me, too. Characteristics and emotions that I deemed undesirable were tucked away, unseen and unacknowledged. Once I began to let others see into me, my homework was to be more intimate with myself and to look farther into this dark side.

Later that week, I reread a journal entry I'd written about a year before I started seeing Iben. In the passage, I describe a dream about my birth family. I found it interesting that our family dynamics were clearly laid out in my subconscious. But what jumped out from the page for me was my sense of superiority and indignation as I analyzed the dream. I felt superior in my capacity for giving and loving, and I was angry with my family for not reciprocating.

When I was telling Iben about the dream, she sat listening silently with her hands open in her lap. Afterward, she said you could sit quietly with the light within your hands or all around you, and in this position others could come to you and receive what they want. Then, she leaned forward and extended her hands closer and closer to me, and I automatically leaned in the opposite direction. She explained that when you try to push your light toward others, they get uncomfortable and move away. She said that righteousness is the need to feel superior and get others to accept your view of reality. She asserted that when you have insight, it is especially easy to fall into the trap of righteousness.

After my layer of righteousness had been peeled away, my homework was to look even deeper into the dark sides of me. I didn't want to do it, but I did, and over the next week some of my dark characteristics showed up in full, naked view: defiance of personal boundaries, superiority, and self-centeredness.

Motivations

Soon after my dark sides were revealed to me, I found a self-description I'd written for school when I was seventeen. I was surprised to find on that page almost every issue I had uncovered with Jackie and Iben! I seemed to have had an awareness of the patterns in my life even at that young age. But something was missing: As a teenager, I'd had no awareness of my own role in creating the dynamics I was experiencing.

Iben gave me her perspective on this new discovery. She said that our world is made up of equal and opposite energies: love, which expands, and fear, which constricts. As part of this natural world, each of us has equal parts of these dual energies. Growing in awareness is developing the ability to choose from which side we will act. Integrity is defined as knowing where you are coming from, taking responsibility for it, and owning the consequences of those actions. She explained that seeing the patterns in your life is often the first step in becoming self-aware, and many people work with a psychologist to gain this type of insight. She said I was in a particularly painful place because I had been aware of the patterns for a long time but they kept repeating. I hadn't gone to the second step, which was appreciating my underlying motivations. I had no awareness of my part in making the issues and situations come back to me over and over again.

Throughout my life, I have often acted from a place of fear without even realizing it, in part because I had no idea of the emotional baggage I was carrying and how it affected my actions. Because I couldn't see my part in creating the dynamics, I often felt like a victim when negative things flowed back to me. After hearing a litany of my work stories when we were young, my husband would marvel that I often threw out grenades and then wondered why I was being attacked. Sometimes, it would suddenly dawn on me that I had acted from a dark place, and I'd usually flush with shame and hide it, deny it, or blame someone else.

As I started to become more aware of my darker side, I could see when my motivations came from this place, and I started to take responsibility when negative stuff flowed back to me. Seeing my part in the dynamics also made me feel more in control and less fearful. I suspected that this helped decrease the tension in my pelvic floor, where I often braced myself, waiting for an inevitable assault.

Hitting Granite

When I first started to work with Iben, she told me that as we went deeper, we would sometimes hit penetrable layers, like soapstone or limestone, and sometimes hit granite. Two months into our work together, I began to hit granite. I must have been ready to unravel those buried issues in my life, because over the next two months, information that helped to clarify those parts of myself came to me from many sources. Information flowed in through my work with Iben as well as from new experiences, dreams, and long-forgotten memories that suddenly resurfaced.

Religion and Me

On Christmas Eve of my second year of pelvic pain, my husband, my children, and I joined the crowd in the school gym for Mass. As usual, I was enjoying the music, the people, and the connection to my past. But as the priest said the opening prayers, I suddenly thought, *This no longer fits me.*

What no longer resonated with me was the idea that I needed an intermediary to connect with God. My connection with God over the past two painful years had come not through the church but rather, more directly, from experiences in my own heart and mind, from the words and actions of people around me, and from nature.

In the service, I also heard the message that I was inherently broken and sinful. While it is true that as I'd probed deeper I'd uncovered the dark sides of me, I had also discovered a lot of light and love within me, too. When I started to uncover my constricting fear-based beliefs and behavior patterns, I could decide whether or not I wanted to continue them. When

I became more aware of my underlying motivations, I had the option of choosing more loving and expanding thoughts and actions.

I felt like a diamond and as though I were cleaning off different facets of myself so the beauty of my inner being could shine forth more brightly. A part of me had always bristled at the thought that I was inherently bad and needed to be saved from myself. As a little girl in Catholic Mass, I never would say the phrase, "Lord, I am not worthy to receive you, but only say the word and I shall be healed." I distinctly remember kneeling in church and thinking, *I am worthy!*

After the Christmas service, my family fully expected to be the last individuals to exit the church because that was my pattern. But that night, I hustled them out before the last notes were sung. As we ran to our car to beat the rush out of the parking lot, my husband laughed and teased, "Who are you?"

Early the next morning, on Christmas Day, I had another Technicolor movie dream. It began with my parents complaining to me about a house they had just bought. It wasn't what they wanted, but they resigned themselves to living with it. Then, the phone rang. On the line was an authority telling me they were going to take care of the problem that very day. I started to cry in gratitude; I couldn't believe it was happening so fast. My parents were not so sure it was a good thing, but the horde of engineers and construction workers descended, anyway. When they were done, only two ancient, ivy-covered stone walls stood on a solid-rock foundation.

Then, the scene switched to a bedroom dormer that had been making its way into my dreams for the past few months. In my dreams, this dormer was always at a forty-five–degree angle, and whenever I walked through it, it would wobble and shake.

Next, in this dream, I was treading water in the ocean directly under the dormer. Suddenly, the dormer crashed down on top of me, but I was perfectly fine. Then, I noticed my mother beside me in the water. "I'm free!" she said and tried to swim away. But she sank, and I rescued her. Three times she broke free and sank, and three times I dove down and retrieved her. Finally, I told her I couldn't do it anymore and let go. Others swam in and took care of her.

I woke up smiling, knowing I had just let go of something really big.

At my next session with Iben, I told her I thought the house represented me and I was clearing out what wasn't true to my basic nature. Iben agreed, saying the dream signified the letting go of the structure and dogma of my upbringing.

My religion was definitely part of my personal history. My parents and I had gone to Mass every Sunday, even on vacations, as well as on holy days, first Fridays, and on national holidays for good measure, and I had attended Catholic grade school, high school, and college. But in college and when I relocated to California for my first job, I'd rarely attended church. On one of their first visits to California after I moved away, I could see my parents in the rear-view mirror giving each other suspicious looks as I got lost on the way to Mass. I'd returned to the church only when I had my own kids, and then I'd taught Sunday school, enrolled them in Catholic school, and took them to church each Sunday. Now, I had the sudden realization that I'd pursued Catholicism only when it was linked with family obligation.

When we were talking about the dream, Iben explained that water and the ocean can represent emotion. She also suggested that it was through the structure of the church that I'd connected emotionally with my mother. This was so true. Even as a toddler, I liked sitting next to my mother in church. Physical tenderness was rare in my home, but in that sanctuary, she often held my hand to keep me quiet. I never saw her display strong emotion, either positive or negative, but sometimes my mother would tear up during Mass and I'd watch her.

One time when I was four, I yelled out for no apparent reason just as the host (the unleavened bread considered to be the embodiment of Jesus Christ) was raised up for quiet adoration. My mother grabbed my hand and pulled me down the aisle and then into the darkness of the janitor's closet. She brought her face close to mine and whispered ferociously, "This is the most sacred part of the Mass!" I had never seen her so furious.

Now, with Iben's help, it became clear to me that I'd been wearing my religion, in part, to connect emotionally with my mother.

My Mother and Me

A few weeks later, in mid-January of 2010, I entered my session with Iben and told her I had experienced an emotional reaction the night before that just didn't make sense to me. When my friend Kelly told me she'd gone away for the weekend with some female friends, jealousy and fear of abandonment immediately rose up within me. I was surprised at the emotions, because even though I really liked Kelly, we weren't that close.

Iben said this was probably significant. She told me to close my eyes and replay the situation in my mind. Then, she asked me what I was feeling. To my surprise, after being pain-free for weeks, my exact pelvic pain resurfaced; my bladder hurt.

Iben asked me to close my eyes again and to imagine my pain with a shape, color, and location in my body. It was like watching a little movie playing behind my eyes. I wasn't actively creating it, yet there it was in full view. I could see my pain as a brown, gelatinous capsule sitting horizontally in my lower abdomen.

Iben asked me to become little Mary Ruth and to go inside the capsule. I could see a sad little me sitting in there.

"She left," I said. "She was here but she's gone."

"Who is that?" Iben asked.

"My mother."

After a time, Iben asked, "What are you doing?"

"I'm running around in here and having a tantrum!"

"Can you find a way out of there?"

Try as I might, the thick elastic walls held me in. But after a while, I cut a vertical slit in the brown membrane and slipped outside.

"Where are you now?" Iben asked.

I told her I was sitting in a space in the lower abdomen, and when I looked up I saw membranous walls of yellow, orange, and red surrounding me.

"She was here, but she's gone again," I said.

I sat waiting in that space for a while, until Iben asked me if I could find a way out. It took a while, but I eventually figured out I could climb up the front of the internal abdomen and crawl into the umbilical area. I slowly made my way through a constricting, brown passageway and finally squeezed out.

Iben again asked me where I was. I told her I was in a green, grassy meadow surrounded by steep, snow-capped mountains with a bright blue sky and fluffy white clouds overhead.

"Where is your mother?" Iben asked.

"She's up in the mountains."

"Do you want to ask her if she wants to come down and be with you?"

"No. She's fine up there. Plus, I'm having fun."

"What are you doing?" she asked.

"I'm running, running, running!"

My eyes squinted, and Iben asked me what was happening.

"Oh, the sun is just so bright," I said.

Then, my eyes relaxed. "Okay, the clouds came over and it's better now."

I opened my eyes, and Iben and I sat there beaming at each other.

"Consider this your rebirth," Iben said.

Remembering

The next week, I found a description of me that was written by my mother for an assignment in my senior year of high school. I remember reading her letter as I was sitting at my small desk in the middle of the classroom. I flushed with embarrassment, and I wanted to quickly rip it up to hide the evidence that I was unlovable.

When I read my mother's letter to Kelly and then to Iben, their eyes widened. Iben said that even though she knew my mother through our work together, she was stunned. Both of them told me that the words reflected management and judgment and little compassion. Throughout my life, I'd wanted my mother's love so badly and thought I had to be perfect to win it. Sometimes, I'd praise myself, hoping for a nod or agreement, but she would usually respond with a comment meant to check an inflated ego.

My mother and I were very different. She was active, kept an emotional distance, and exuded control. I was sedentary, emotional, open, and physically demonstrative—qualities that were not really seen nor valued in my childhood home.

A clear memory of one of my last visits home to see my mother surfaced, and I told Iben about it. I'd driven from the airport to my hometown and met my sister for lunch. As we were eating our burgers, we heard a siren and both said, "That might be Mom." She was suffering from ALS and breast cancer and had been in hospice care for two weeks. After quickly finishing our lunch, we decided to check the hospital in town before driving to her home, twenty minutes away. We found her in the emergency room, bleeding internally. The doctor said her blood level was so low it was incompatible with life, so he ordered two blood transfusions for her.

Later, my mom told me she felt so poorly at that point that she'd thought it was the end. During the blood transfusions, we were alone in her treatment room, and she asked me to lean in close so she could tell me something. I thought this might be the moment when, finally, she told me she loved me. Instead, she whispered that her friend, who was also her private nurse, had been so helpful that she wanted to make sure to thank her properly. She wanted her friend to come to California for a vacation with me, and she would pay for it. I had waited my whole life to connect with my mother, and it was disappointing to think those may have been our final words.

Later that week, as my mother watched television, almost motionless in her recliner after having made it through two blood transfusions, I mustered up the courage to ask the question that had been burning inside me. "Mom, do you love me?"

She wondered out loud why I didn't know that. She told me to think of how much I loved my own children and then to consider that she held the same feelings for her own kids.

Then, I asked, "Have I met your expectations as a daughter?"

"You have done everything perfect your whole life," she replied.

The sentiments were nice, but I was yearning for intimacy and unconditional love.

Really Looking

The week after I told Iben this story, I had a dream that my mother died and I was attending an impromptu gathering at the church. My mother's friends were telling stories of how close she was to them, and one woman was just inconsolable. Then, my mom appeared at the side of the table. I told her I needed to be hugged or told I was loved. But then I felt bad; it seemed wrong to bring up my issues when she was the one who had just died. At that point, a man came over and told me they needed help with the autopsy, which was being performed in the corner of the church. I thought, *Why is it always me?*

In the next scene of my dream, I sat at the head of the table holding on to a glass canister full of my mother's breath while particles of smoke engulfed and choked me. I looked down to see her dead body with a gaping maw and all the brains inside. I decided not to look again. Then, the spirit of an older woman holding a discontented baby rose up. I didn't recognize the woman's face, but her eyes were definitely my mother's, and I knew I was the frowning baby. I looked up and said, "I love you, Mom." She stumbled over it the first time but then told me she loved me, too. She ascended, up and away.

Iben said the dream signified the difficulty I had with looking honestly at my mother.

I replied, "How can you be mad at a saint?"

My mother was generous, insightful, genuinely interested in others, and the best listener you could meet. At her funeral, the priest said she was a true disciple of Jesus in action, and almost fifty people nodded in agreement.

I started to appreciate how difficult it had been to reconcile my feelings of being hurt and not supported by my mom with the fact that she was this great, benevolent woman. I had spent a lifetime carrying around anger and disappointment and then berating myself for feeling that way.

Throughout my life, I stored up memories of my mother's perceived failings and often complained about her. This never led to any healing or resolution for me. Now, I was looking at our relationship again but from a different vantage point. Instead of focusing on her, I focused on how our relationship had impacted me. Looking at my own feelings and reactions was painful, and I knew my mother would have considered this type of analysis to be self-indulgent.

Faced with these thoughts and feelings, I started to shy away from looking further into this relationship with my mother, but Iben encouraged me to continue. She explained that this relationship colored my whole world when I was a child; it had been my reality. As an adult, those experiences were reflected in my inner voice.

I had spent a lifetime ruminating over issues with my mother, but once I really looked at them, their hold on my heart and mind started to melt away. Over time, I began to see my mother as another soul on this journey of life, with her own challenges and triumphs, her own light and dark sides, and her own inner voice—just like me. As my compassion for myself grew, I began to have a lot more compassion for my mother, too.

Cellular Memory

Iben explained that sometimes pain is a message from the body, like a GPS signaling me that I'm a bit off-course. At other times, this discomfort is a flare-up of cellular memory. She went on to explain that experiences and belief systems are stored at the cellular level, like data on a computer's hard drive. This information runs much like programs, and some can create imbalance and cause physical symptoms in the body. Iben said that her work (called cellular memory reprogramming) identifies areas in the body where this cellular memory is stored and aids in releasing it, and this helps restore balance and promote wellness.

Before my pain began, this idea of cellular memory reprogramming would have sounded ridiculous to me. Now, it was difficult to fully deny it, because after I'd done the work with Iben related to the relationship with my mother, my bladder pain went away and did not return for a full year.

The Feminine Connection

After I worked through some of the relationship issues with my mother, my history with women rose to the forefront of my mind, and I told Iben about it. For as far back as I could remember, I'd never felt comfortable with women, and most of my significant relationships in the past had been with men.

Every single year from kindergarten through ninth grade, I met a nice girlfriend and invested time with her, only for her family to move away the following year. Often, groups of girls would ban together and push me out in aggressive ways. For example, at a high school graduation party, a group of "friends" sat in a circle and proceeded to tell me what was wrong with me. When I left the circle, went into another part of the room, and laid face-down on the carpet sobbing, they surrounded me again and continued the assault. Experiences like this played out over and over again—with neighborhood girls, with middle school classmates, twice in college, and even once on my very first job.

This disconnection with women had not inherently changed in adulthood and with my illness. When I was in the peak of pain, my neighbor Lee had held me like a mother, but then I hadn't heard from her again for a full year. Even my daughter, Katherine, at age fifteen, had little connection with and compassion for what I was going through. Once, she told me I didn't have any friends, and she was right.

Iben helped me to look deeper at the hurts I was carrying with regard to my relationships with women and to appreciate my contribution to the dynamics I was experiencing. I have always been a loving, giving person, but along with that had come an intense need to be filled up, to be validated and loved back. All that positive energy flowing out of me was accompanied by an undercurrent of emotional need that could push people away. Iben explained that yin energy is similar to female sexuality in that it accepts love and flows it back. In my relationships with women, I was often more like yang (male) energy, and the more I pushed for connection, the more women backed off. I had no faith that love would find me if I didn't try to get it with all my effort.

My journal shows that I was now willing to connect with women:

> My inner voice called out, "I want to have girlfriends!" And another inner voice called back, "They are coming, be patient."

After this healing and over time, women would step closer and closer to me and invite me into their groups and lives. I now have close relationships with my neighbors, Lee and Kelly, and with my daughter. Katherine often comments that I have a lot of friends and many of them are women—and she's right!

More Awareness, More Granite

At this point during my work with Iben, my symptoms changed. I no longer had the bladder pain, and the deep pelvic-floor muscles were no longer in spasm. But then, the superficial pelvic-floor muscles that surround the opening of the vagina and rectum started to spasm. For about a year, I also had recurrent vaginal bacterial infections. I was scared these new symptoms were the start of a new pain condition.

I started receiving physical therapy treatments from Julie again, and she encouraged me to remain calm and just ride it out. Iben suggested I look within and determine specifically what the fear was about. Then, I should just allow the fear to be and transfer the emotional energy into thoughts or actions that would further my growth.

The week after Iben made that suggestion, I had a dream. I was looking through the eyes of my higher self, which was positioned near the ceiling and studying another version of myself sitting at a table in the real world. My lower self looked up and our eyes met. It was so obvious how scared the lower self was! As the higher self, I flowed out love and encouragement, and I could feel others standing in support behind me. Then, the lower self disappeared, and as I woke up, the two parts of me merged into one.

The Home Front

After Iben and I had addressed the issues with my mother, I started to focus on my relationship with my husband, as evidenced by this journal entry:

> *Alex is so independent, and it hurts me when he doesn't connect with me. I try to be charming, and he makes little snippy jokes. I like to be spontaneous, and he considers it just a bother. We haven't been walking at night. He is busy, preoccupied, and he will be traveling next week. I'm*

feeling alone, like I am not connected with others. I'm feeling needy, like I have to grab or entertain to get what I need.

At my next session with Iben after writing that in my journal, the first thing I said upon entering the treatment room was, "There are a lot of parallels between the relationship with my mom and the relationship with my husband."

Iben shared with me that she was surprised and pleased that I was entering that awareness. She said that dynamic had been clear to her from the first day we met, but she hadn't mentioned it because, at the time, my relationship with Alex was holding me together. Now that I was starting to understand myself better, I was no longer defined by my relationship with my husband nor enmeshed in our dynamics. From this separate vantage point, the patterns of our partnership came into view, and I wondered, really wondered, *Why did I turn on the lights!*

Iben said that when someone gains awareness, the change affects the people and relationships surrounding that person. She described it like a small crack in a windshield that expands and spreads outward.

My massage therapist, Chris, said it was like Alex and I had been dancing the tango for over two decades, and then I began dancing the rumba. Before, our steps may not have been perfectly healthy, but they were well practiced. Now, everything seemed uncoordinated, and we were stepping on each other's toes a lot.

Both Dr. Ryan and Dr. Noblett questioned me about my home situation, and they both made links between my new physical symptoms and the issues I was uncovering in my marriage. Once again, I was reminded of the connection between the physical and emotional parts of me. So I was motivated to look at the relationship issues with my husband that I was carrying, because uncovering and understanding those issues was a possible way out of my physical discomfort.

Marital Hierarchy

As mentioned earlier in this chapter, through my work with Iben I became aware of my disdain for hierarchy, especially when I felt I was in a subordinate role. How surprising and frustrating it was to realize that I had recreated that dynamic in my marriage!

Alex is the oldest of five children, and I'm the youngest of four, so we easily fell into the roles of him as the big brother and me as the youngest sibling. No matter how accomplished I was or how much respect he had for me, he was in charge and I was the underling. That also was the theme of almost every one of his jokes. I completely participated in this dynamic, and in my mind, I put him up on a pedestal and me in an inferior role.

Iben explained that at age fifty many men are in the "king" stage of development. They see everything they do as serving the family. They provide for the castle, fix the castle, make sure the castle is safe, and so on. The king also wants the queen to be happy—or at least to look and act as if everything is in order—and he wants the prince and princess to do well, too.

I started to tease Alex by calling him "king" but stopped when I realized he actually liked the title.

Iben said it was good for Alex to be king, but I needed to step up into my position as queen and set boundaries when I did not receive the respect I deserved in our home.

Projects and People

Alex is a project person, and he almost always chooses to complete a project over connecting with people. Before my illness, I was a project person, too. Early in our marriage, Alex had to complain for a full week and then blow up before I would stop working so we could go get a Christmas tree. After we had been together for eight years, it was Alex who began pushing me to start a family. I kept putting it off because I was focused on teaching and research.

But through my internal work, I realized that achievement was my way to get acceptance and love. For me, connecting with others was always a huge underlying motivation for my work.

I also realized that the lack of emotional connection in my life had always been a source of discontent. I silently resented when others did not meet my emotional needs, and I held those feelings tightly within. For example, on our honeymoon over twenty years ago, I'd planned a trip up the California coast with stays at quaint bed and breakfasts. Engaging in romantic conversations on the beach and visiting with strangers in close quarters just wasn't Alex's style. So he'd decided to cut the trip short, and we spent the week working on our new home. I went along with the plan and buried my disappointment that the honeymoon had not met my romantic expectations.

Emotional Connection

Iben often described the right side of the body (controlled by the left hemisphere of the brain) as the male side and the left side of the body (controlled by the right hemisphere of the brain) as the female side. From this perspective, no one is better at meeting right-sided needs than Alex. He is a traditional male. The right side is where he lives and breathes and what he values. It would be difficult to find a better provider and protector.

For the first twenty-five years of our relationship, the right side of me was the only part that was developed. But when the internal work I was doing allowed the left/feminine side of me to emerge more, I found it to be a huge part of who I am. And it was starving for emotional and physical tenderness! I also knew it was easy to focus on the side with needs, and if I had emotional and physical tenderness but didn't feel well provided for, that would be a problem, too.

It had become clear to me that Alex and I were very different at a basic level. He dealt with the world from an intellectual and physical standpoint, and I often came from an emotional perspective. When our conversations would veer in an emotional direction, Alex would usually thwart them with humor, interrupt me, or change the subject. When I tried to give and receive more emotional or physical tenderness, he would often get irritated and say he felt controlled. I would chase Alex for connection, and he would put up boundaries.

Iben explained that Alex and I both had individual emotional needs, and what he needed most was for me to have no emotional needs. She joked that Alex wanted a "Stepford wife" with substance. When I shared Iben's joke with Alex, he laughed and said, "That would be nice!"

A New Perspective

Iben gave me different ways to look at my marriage so that I would feel empowered to have the life I envisioned. Here are some of her suggestions:

- Accept that it is what it is.
- Picture Alex and me as equal partners with two bodies and four legs walking next to each other.
- Consider that Alex gives presents in the form of service and action rather than in the form of emotional presence. See the service he provides as the way he says, "I love you," and appreciate the gifts he gives to me in my life.
- Consider how life would be if Alex were emotionally needy. Picture him leaning on me, and figure out whether that is what I really wanted.
- Have no expectations for intense emotional connection with Alex, because at that point, he doesn't tap into his emotions or express them. Iben said that in her experience people grow emotionally but do not change fundamentally unless they choose that path themselves and work on it.
- Meet my own needs to connect with others, and imagine myself being surrounded by relationships that meet my emotional needs. Iben explained that one person could not meet all my needs and that I could be surrounded by loving, emotional connections without forsaking my relationship with Alex.

Spinning and the Spiral

One week when the marital dynamics between Alex and me were especially painful, I felt like I was spinning. My inner voice was fearful and judging, and I started to push myself. My bladder pain resurfaced.

I asked Iben, "Do you think I'm just completely overwhelmed, or do you think I'm regrouping and growing?"

"You can be both at the same time," she replied.

She went on to say that I didn't have any support that week, and my body was trying to hold itself together. Once again, she asked me to consider switching my perspective toward my body from one of fear and frustration with the pain to one of gratitude that my body was telling me something.

At that point, I was starting to become aware of the main patterns in my life, and sometimes, I knew what it actually felt like to be grounded or centered. But just when I'd start to feel settled and peaceful, one of my common issues would pop up and send my mind spinning again. It was discouraging, and I'd think, *Not this one again. I thought I had moved past this!* I wondered if I were moving forward only to fall right back to my starting point. Then, I noticed that the same issues in my life seemed to be coming around more often, and I wondered if I were regressing.

Iben described spiritual progression as being like a spiral that moves in an upward direction and gets smaller and smaller in diameter as it ascends. The same issues come around again and again, but each time they are revisited from a higher vantage point and experienced with greater awareness. As we ascend spiritually in this way, the patterns and experiences in life come around quicker and quicker.

The goal of spiritual growth, Iben explained, is not to become devoid of feelings or to have no reaction to life; it is to become more open and aware, to fully experience life and one's humanness. As you grow spiritually, the highs and lows actually become even more intense because you are more conscious of your thoughts, emotions, and body reactions. What changes as you grow in awareness is that you stay more centered within yourself during the experience and can see the experience as separate from who you are. It no longer defines you.

9

A New Place

A few months after I started working with Iben and after two and a half years of various other treatments, the pain in my bladder and pelvic-floor muscles subsided. Although I was feeling good physically, I continued to work on a weekly basis with Iben for nine more months to address emotional and spiritual issues. For a full year in 2010, I lived relatively pain-free and no longer needed appointments with my caregivers. I walked into a peaceful place on this journey and was able to rest, reflect, and connect further with my inner self.

The Healing Power of Human Connection

After my father died, my cousin Rich called to offer his condolences. I shared with him how difficult it had been for me to say goodbye to all the people in my hometown whom I held in my heart and that I felt such a sense of loss. He asked me to clarify who I was talking about, and after I did, he said, "Oh, your parents' friends—their people." Upon hearing these words, I suddenly realized I was holding on to the connections my parents had made more than twenty years before, thousands of miles away, because I had so few of my own.

Likewise, when I saw the apes lounging around at the zoo, I saw parallels to my life. I longed to be in the middle of the grooming circle, but I was often the lone monkey observing the proceedings from some distant rock. But after working through my deeper issues during the years of pain, I started to step into the inner circle of connection.

Connection and Community

My journal entry written in late 2009, right before I started seeing Iben, shows my yearning to be part of a community:

> I heard on the radio today that we all have a natural need to be part of a community, and I know that's true for me. When I grew up, many of our family activities were centered around a close-knit community and church. But I don't miss the competition and not being able to be just me. I tried to be a part of the local church for years with the kids, but the community wasn't a warm one. So I miss being part of a group, and I can develop this over time with people of like mind.

For years, my massage therapist, Chris, encouraged me to become part of a community. She suggested I check out the Unitarian Universalist church near my house because it welcomed all faiths and encouraged the individual's own spiritual journey. The night before I attended my first service at the church she had recommended, I had a dream in which I was sitting alone in the church, surrounded by people I didn't know, happy and smiling.

My neighbor Lee was planning to go with me, but I wasn't surprised when she came to the door in her pajamas, having forgotten about our date. I knew I'd be going alone on that first day because I'd been alone in my dream.

I began regularly attending church services, discussion groups, and choir. I was connecting with a community, and this time it was mine.

Gauging Personal Growth

The second service I attended wasn't a traditional one, and members were reading fairy tales to the group as part of an exploration of story and myth. Bob was the first reader. He was eighty-six at the time, tall and slim, with slicked-back white hair and intense blue eyes darting over his Roman nose. Through his voice, the characters came alive and danced around in my imagination.

Afterward, I approached Bob in the courtyard and told him how much I'd enjoyed his reading.

He retorted, "Well, I didn't write it!"

"I know you didn't write it, but you did a great job reading it."

"Well, I should have. I've worked as an actor and director my whole life." He scoffed at me like an underling trying to get a part.

I looked at him directly and said, "Do you have trouble taking compliments?"

"Well, praise is a lot like filling up on cotton candy. I want it, but it does me no good later."

He started to talk about directing, and I picked up on the parallels between our jobs. His description of drawing out the inherent potential in an actor was very similar to the process I used as a physical therapist when I helped patients relearn how to move after suffering a stroke.

Partway through our conversation, Bob's eyes sparkled and he exclaimed, "*You* should be a director!"

When I told Iben about this interaction, she laughed and said, "People can be like messengers. You are dealing with a hierarchical male in your home, and Bob is giving you practice with this dynamic without all the emotional attachment."

My interactions also helped me gauge where I was in my own healing. For example, before my illness, I would have cowered at Bob's initial prickliness, and anytime he was near, I would have tightened up with fear of being hurt. But through the challenge of my illness, I had grown more solid and centered, and now I could stand up and look Bob right in the eye. We both liked the challenge, and our friendship grew. Over time, our relationship became sustaining and healing for both of us.

Colors of Connection

I noticed that when I was with certain people, my pelvic-floor muscles were often completely relaxed. The people who had this healing effect on me were diverse. Old and young, female and male, they came from all walks of life, and I met them in different places in my life. Some were old friends with whom I now shared a deeper relationship—like Lee and Kelly, both of whom I had known for over twenty years. Some were new acquaintances and friends.

I met one of my new friends, Jeff, in a physical therapy clinic where he was working as an aide and I was rehabilitating a foot injury. We bonded quickly, and he would often stay through lunch to continue a conversation we'd started on the treatment table. Even though we were different genders and twenty years apart, we had similar interpersonal and learning styles, career interests, and emotional/spiritual experiences. Once Jeff and I sat on a bench at the beach and talked for five straight hours, neither of us noticing the sunburns we were incurring at the time. You can count the number of spiritual books I've read on one hand, but Jeff has been reading them for years. When I told him about my personal experiences, he often validated them and put them in a larger perspective.

Before then, my main socialization had been with my children and husband. Now, I was developing close connections outside of my home.

I worried that spending time and energy on developing friendships with other people would negatively impact my marriage and family. When I relayed those concerns to Iben, she explained that love is like pure white light, and when this light goes through a prism, it separates into different colors. In the same way, each of my relationships had its own unique hue of loving connection.

The morning after Iben shared that analogy with me, I woke up with a clear image of my body superimposed with a rainbow of colors. It looked just like pictures I've seen of chakras. Developed in Hinduism and Buddhism, chakras depict the seven major energy centers of the body through which life energy is considered to flow into and out of a person. Each chakra emits an aura (invisible but detectable energy) that is associated with a specific color and meaning. For example, Chakra One, located at the base of the spine and represented by the color red, is associated with one's physical identity and self-preservation (health, prosperity, security, stability, etc.).

Along with the image of my body superimposed with chakras of different colors came the realization that my relationships all had individual hues that matched the colors of my being. For example, my relationship with Jeff was characterized by indigo between the brows, representing spiritual insight (the third eye), and blue at the neck, representing communication. My relationship with my husband, Alex, was primarily red at the tailbone (the root), representing my survival and my family. In this way, each of my connections was unique, and all of them in combination nourished my whole person.

I found that when I allowed myself to be filled up with loving interactions in my life, it didn't take away from my family. I actually had more to bring to them.

As Iben said, "When it is love, it grows . . . and love creates more love."

My Body, My Messenger

Over the year I worked with Iben, the messages from my body became more specific, intense, and instantaneous, and I began to use this information more often in my life. If my mind said, *I'm fine with this*, but my pelvic-floor muscles went into a spasm, that physical reaction almost always revealed my truth. Iben said the mind has prior conditioning and can deceive you, but the body doesn't lie.

If I were contemplating which action to take, sometimes I would think about my different options, and after each one, my pelvic floor would either tense up or relax. I had no idea that this body response would become more obvious, specific, and useful in the years to come. When I was going through a particularly stressful time or working through an issue, a sensation of fullness in the bladder would occasionally resurface. In the past, this would have frightened me. But now I knew my body was telling me something. My friend Jeff told me my body was now an internal GPS that told me when I was off-course.

Sitting on the Side of the Road

Before the pain began, I used to slug down my coffee as I entered the gym, and while I was exercising on the machines, I would listen to my blaring iPod, watch TV, and study for my physical therapy classes, sometimes all at the same time. Now, I just exercise and time passes peacefully. I also prefer to walk in nature and do yoga rather than spend time in the noisy gym. I used to read a magazine or study whenever I was in a waiting room. Now, I often just sit quietly. I used to listen to negative talk radio or loud music whenever I was home alone. Now, I enjoy silence or inspirational music. I used to spend lots of time shopping and watching television. Now, I'd rather write, sing, or visit with a friend.

Although chronic pain kept me on the sidelines of my life for years, sitting on the side of the road for so long gave me a new perspective. Today, that new perspective keeps me grounded as others rush past. What was once a forced state is now my chosen state.

Iben said that, in the past, I was "being through doing"—a way of living that is highly valued in my family and culture. Then, during my healing process, I began to experience "doing through being." Iben explained that every person is a unique creation; there is only one of each of us. When you are aligned with your true being, it can be a great gift to the world, no matter which actions you undertake at the time. If you focus on being productive or busy, you connect with others when you find the time. In contrast, if you are just "being," you are much more available for real connections.

After giving Iben's explanation some thought, it occurred to me that when I was "being through doing," I was using the activity to define or validate myself. When I was "doing through being," my actions were a joyful expression of my inner person.

To experience this new state of being and to appreciate my inner person, I needed a break from constant activity. In fact, I had to be pulled off my life for years in order to reset my pace from manic to harmonic—in tune with my body, mind, and spirit. Once that happened, instead of rushing around, I could often be fully present in my life, going with the flow and sometimes just pausing to be.

Inner Peace

For almost fifty years, I criticized my body and I scrutinized and managed my thoughts and emotions. It was like an internal war zone! Now, that negative, driving voice within is usually replaced by a loving and compassionate one. Whereas I used to be entrenched in my mind and almost completely cut off from the signals of my body and emotions, now all parts of me often chime in. My body, mind, and emotions usually keep me aware of what I'm experiencing or processing in the moment, and I often have a sense of inner peace.

This state of being is sometimes described as being awake, aware, or conscious. At one time, I thought these words were just New Age propaganda. Indeed, when I first read Eckhart Tolle's description of this state of mind, I thought it was just his individual response to severe depression. But now I had experienced a little bit of how it feels to experience life from this vantage point.

"It is so interesting," I told Iben. "The answers are within. You just have to open up and become aware of them."

Beaming at me, Iben said, "Yes, it really is quite simple."

The Healing Mind–Spirit Connection

At the beginning of my illness when I wondered whether I would ever be better, my caregivers encouraged me to envision and set my sights on recovery. They knew that the mind-body connection was powerful.

Two and a half years into my pain, I met Catherine outside my physical therapist's office, and we talked for two hours. She was another messenger on this healing road, an intimate stranger meant just for me. Catherine told me about her connection with nature during her struggle to survive stage-four breast cancer. She went on to tell me that in waiting rooms she could often tell which patients had given up and which were digging deep. She said she felt an inherent power within and used it to survive, and she asked me to write about it to let others know it was possible. When Catherine told me about this power she felt, I thought it was a nice sentiment but I wasn't sure it was true. But six months later when I landed in this peaceful place, Catherine's words resounded in my ears.

At about that time, I sheepishly admitted to my friend Christine that I was starting to have more confidence in my ability to alter the course of events in my body. In response, Christine, a ten-year survivor of stage-three breast cancer, told me her story. When initially diagnosed, she'd cornered her doctor and pushed him to reveal her odds of survival. When he'd said she had less than a twenty percent chance of surviving five years, she'd gone home stunned and devastated. But then, standing in her bedroom, she'd felt a deep resounding resolve from her very core, asserting, *This will not be!* Christine made it clear to me that this thought wasn't something superficial coming from her mind as a way to get what she wanted. It felt much deeper than that, like it was coming from her soul. She also said that willing yourself better may not be in line with the needs of your soul or the plans of God, so it may not always happen.

In these dire circumstances, both of these women felt they had tapped into the creative, healing power of their souls. This encouraged me. Perhaps my new ideas weren't totally crazy!

Gratitude for Growth

At my one-year anniversary of working with Iben, I reread my journal entry written the night after our first visit, in which I'd summarized her first impressions:

- *My spirit did not fully enter my body at birth. . . . I often lived my life through others, and I hadn't fully experienced my own body and my own life.*
- *. . . I'd had a glimpse of being centered but hadn't fully landed yet.*
- *In the past, I didn't love without expectation, and that's why it didn't always flow back. Accompanying this loving energy were neediness and fear of abandonment, and these thoughts and emotions helped create negative relationships and experiences in my life.*
- *Intense resentment that is not expressed often goes to the bladder (literally, being pissed off) . . .*
- *. . . .I am very intuitive. . . .*
- *I am mostly yin (female) energy, and my mom was mostly yang (male) energy.*
- *. . . my body was moving to become grounded and was turning me to the left, the feminine side.*
- *I have a low libido.*
- *"When you are aligned with who you think you should be rather than with whom you truly are, the body will try to call you back to center."*

When I read through this list, I started to laugh. I couldn't believe Iben had picked up my main issues on that very first visit. Of course, hearing her words didn't mean that I immediately and fully understood, believed, and worked through these issues. Although Iben had given me an outline of the issues to be addressed and a preview of what my journey might entail, I still had to go through the process of coming to those realizations and working through them on my own and in my own time. She could show me the dirt, but I needed to get down there and crawl through it.

Frankly, I was extremely skeptical after that first visit, because the language and concepts Iben used were so foreign to me. In fact, they were completely different than the belief system and social conditioning I had subscribed to for almost fifty years. However, beyond ideas and words was my own tangible experience of opening up in the very core of me, and that was my truth. Over the year of working with Iben, my body became pain-free, my mind quieted, and I watched as the experiences and relationships in my life transformed around me.

I had started this process with Iben as a way to heal my body and get out of physical pain. After mining the depths with her, I realized that my mind and spirit, too, wanted to stop suffering and heal.

On our anniversary visit, I sat cross-legged on Iben's treatment table as she stood by my side in the warm, candle-lit room. Beaming at her, I mused, "Consider where I was just twelve months ago. To be in this place is a miracle."

Why It Worked

Having previously worked for a year and a half with a good psychologist, I was completely surprised by how much more I'd learned about myself with Iben. There are several reasons why I think our collaboration was successful.

Most important, Iben was a good match for me on a personal level. I felt comfortable with her and safe enough to be honest and vulnerable. Incredibly self-aware and intuitive, she was also loving, humble, and human. When I looked at how she lived her life, it was genuine; her actions matched what she was telling me. Iben often had insight into my issues way ahead of me, but she knew how to pace my sessions, pushing me to grow but not revealing so much that I shut down. During our work together, I felt progressively more empowered rather than more dependent.

Sometimes, I left a session questioning or a bit destabilized, but I was never afraid.

These relationship characteristics can be used as a guide when choosing a caregiver who works at the emotional or spiritual levels. As a patient, it is also important to keep your own power, and if the sessions don't meet your needs, don't hesitate to move on.

A Personal Path, Not a Generic Prescription

I told several friends about the work I was doing with Iben and the healing that had resulted from it. Many of them confided that, while they knew my experience was completely valid, they definitely didn't want to go there themselves. I could totally relate, because I'd been forty-five and debilitated with pain before I'd started to look at the stuff I was carrying inside.

My friends' resistance comes partly from their thinking the process may be scary or painful. Sometimes, it *was* very difficult to revisit my emotional pain. But I was carrying the stuff already, and looking at it helped relieve the pressure of the load. The best part was that, once I processed an issue, it no longer weighed me down. Looking at these deeper issues was a bit like exercising: I often dreaded the workout but felt so much lighter and healthier afterward. Like getting in physical shape, the more I looked at my internal issues, the better I felt and the more motivated I was to continue.

What I feared most were change and the unknown, which is probably why I had to suffer so much before I was willing to move out of my comfort zone. But the ability to avoid change is really an illusion. The future is never completely predictable, and I was always changing, whether or not I was consciously aware of it.

A few friends admitted to feeling guilty about resisting this internal work.

"My experiences are just that—*my* experiences. They aren't a prescription for others," I replied. "This is my healing path; it might not be yours. We each get to choose when and how we want to travel."

10

Full Circle

After working so hard for so long, I was proud of having beaten the pain and thrilled about having landed in a healthier place not only physically but also emotionally and spiritually. When I had been pain-free for about a year, I began to feel a little cocky about my hard-won recovery. . . . That's when the pain crept up again!

Suddenly, in January of 2011, my internal and external pelvic muscles started to spasm, and I could feel my nervous system gradually ramping up again. Even the bladder pain made another appearance. The pain level was a three or four on a scale of one to ten, and it bothered me from ten to fifty percent of my day. Although the pain wasn't as intense as when it had appeared the first time around, I was still incredibly annoyed by it and very discouraged it had come back.

Although being completely cured makes for an inspiring story, having an occasional flare-up is much more common for people with chronic conditions, especially pelvic pain. The truth is, even though I like to think of myself as invincible, I am human and vulnerable, and sometimes I hurt. My body has been through a lot and it remembers. We all have weak links where stress settles in and signals us, and the pelvic area is mine.

I realized that life doesn't go in a straight line and it is natural to have peaks and valleys. I'd been in a deep valley for two years, during which I'd gained the insight and strength to reach a pinnacle of well-being that had lasted for almost a year. Then, I entered the valley again, and my symptoms waxed and waned as I worked toward becoming pain-free once again. Just as before, the journey through this valley brought depth to my life. This chapter reveals some of what I learned during my second bout with pelvic pain.

Same Pain, Different Me

Even though the pain returned, I suffered a lot less than I had the first time around. Although I was traveling a similar terrain, I was a different person inside my heart and mind. I was in the desert again, but now I had a well-developed oasis where I could rest and be renewed. Instead of becoming anxious and overly active, I rested and took care of myself. Instead of thinking I would be isolated and lonely and then panicking at that thought, I took comfort in the knowledge that I was lovable and connected to the people around me. When I was hurting, I often rested in meditation and placed my hands over my bladder. My body also frequently moved into spontaneous unwinding, after which I would feel a light tingling throughout my body and my pain level would drop.

Both Pam (my acupuncturist) and Dr. Ryan (my internist and general practitioner) remarked how much calmer I was with the second flare-up than I'd been when the pain had first appeared three and a half years before. They reminisced about the times when I'd cried in their offices, wondering whether I would ever be pain-free again. They said this time was easier on me emotionally because I knew a pain-free state was possible and I knew the way back there. They reminded me that it takes time for things to calm down once they're stirred up, and they encouraged me to be patient.

I tried to listen to their advice, but when the pain hung around for several months and the percentage of time I was hurting each day crept up to eighty percent, I didn't remain calm. At times, I experienced depths of despair similar to what I'd felt at the very beginning of my illness. Sometimes during the second flare-up, I again felt how exhausting and discouraging this journey can be and I felt trapped in my painful body. Any feelings of superiority I may have harbored about how I'd handled my illness the first time around were replaced with compassion for those who were trapped in that hole of suffering. I realized it could easily be me in that same place, and sometimes it is.

I analyzed why the pain had flared up. Just like before, I found that interrelated factors in my body, mind, and spirit had contributed to the pain ramp-up. It was much easier to figure out the underlying issues the second time around because the first journey through the pain had tuned me into all these aspects of myself. My body, mind, and spirit were all very boisterous now!

The Body

First off, for several months I had plantar fasciitis (inflammation of the thick tissue on the bottom of the foot) in my left foot, which tightened my calf muscles and changed my walking pattern. This, in turn, altered the stress on my pelvic-floor muscles and put a noxious input into my nervous system, which may have contributed to the ramp-up of my pelvic pain.

To be honest, the other contributing factor was that I hadn't managed my physical condition for six whole months. I'd stopped watching my diet and working on my internal pelvic muscles, and I rarely did physical exercise or yoga. What was I thinking? After all I had been through, you would think I'd have known better, but I thought I was completely cured and didn't need to take care of myself anymore.

Needless to say, after the pain reared up, I got back on track and started watching my diet, swimming, going to yoga, and doing my exercises to relax and stretch my internal and external pelvic muscles. When the pain didn't resolve after a few weeks, I gradually set up appointments with all of my caregivers. As usual, each professional saw the ramp-up of pain from her own perspective and helped me address that aspect of the overall problem.

The Mind and Spirit

When I saw Iben, she placed her hand over my bladder and said, "You are in a flare-up, and I feel some resentment here."

I told her my mind had been spinning for about a month before the pain began. While we were talking, I recognized my old pattern. I had lost some of the connection to myself and was looking to others to validate me and fill me up. When my chosen targets couldn't meet my emotional needs, I felt cut off, needy, and resentful. I was especially prone to chasing people who were warm and connected sometimes and quiet and withholding at other times. When their response to me vacillated, I would lose my own power and take a subordinate role. I had repeated this pattern with my mother, siblings, husband, and some of my friends.

Iben encouraged me to become more aware of the signs that I was falling into this co-dependent state. The signals for me were a constricting feeling in my pelvic area and the need to share personal stuff at a rapid pace in the hope of impressing people. With this pattern came the tendency to look at others with idealism. In some ways, I was trying to mold them, to give them characteristics that could fill my needs.

Iben told me that people often show who they are within the first or second meeting. Unless a person goes through a transformative growth, that is how he or she will always be and how one's relationship with that person will remain. We revisited my first date with Alex, and lo and behold, our personal qualities and the nature of our relationship were all right there!

Iben explained that when I was realistic, I could accept others for who they were. I could allow them to just be and not pile on expectations for them or for our relationship that couldn't be met.

"People are not in your life to be how you want them to be," she reminded me.

Experiencing this dynamic again made it clearer to me. I no longer saw this side of myself as bad or evil, just as constricting and painful. I actually smiled at the sight of this old, familiar part of me that hadn't been in my life for a while but had wreaked lots of havoc in the past. Once I could see it, I had the opportunity to choose a healthier way for my mind, body, and spirit.

Let's Talk

One morning I woke up to the bladder pain already screaming for my attention. I thought, *Oh, this is going to be a rough day.* I placed my hands over my lower abdomen and laid there with a very quiet mind for about a half hour as I slowly repeated, "I am pain-free. I am pain-free." Suddenly and to my great surprise, the bladder pain stopped. Even though the pain came back later that day, this was a powerful experience for me. Before, I'd often been able to relax my muscles with breathing and calm attention to the area, but I had no idea I could affect the organs in that way.

When I told Julie, my physical therapist, about the experience, she replied, "Oh, yes, you can definitely talk to the organs."

I started to tap into this mind-body connection more often. I would rest in a quiet state with my hands over the bladder and concentrate on sending loving, healing energy to the area. When my pain levels dropped, I would just smile at the fascinating capabilities of the body-mind-spirit.

Family Drama

Our family dynamics had been shifting quite a bit over the past year, and the relationship between Alex and me continued to challenge both of us. We often got caught in our old pattern, in which he would reinforce the old hierarchy and I would hold resentment and anger.

Iben explained that there was a difference between accommodation and compromise, and when I compromised, I made myself smaller. She encouraged me to not "shrink to fit." It became clear to me that when I took that route, it almost always led to suppressed anger and physical pain.

Alex often reverted to our old patterns. Even though my previous work had made me aware of these patterns, I would either fall right into the common dynamic or get frustrated that our relationship wasn't different. Then, five years into my pain, I healed some very deep emotional wounds, which had created patterns in my behavior that affected all the relationships in my life, including my marriage. Only when I realized my contributions to these unhealthy dynamics was I able to stop being an equal and active participant in them. After this personal growth, my interactions with Alex and others close to me felt more positive and peaceful.

Being Sexual

During a treatment a few months into the second flare-up of pain, Iben placed her hands on my lower abdomen right over my bladder, and we both could tell it was distended, stiff, and tender. All my pelvic muscles were also pulled tight.

Iben asked me what percentage of my whole person I felt I was experiencing and expressing in my life. I said about eighty percent. She remarked that not expressing one fifth of me was suppressing quite a bit. She also explained that, anatomically, the pelvic region took up about the same portion of my body—one fifth.

After we talked a while, Iben said I had grown into quite a full being but not yet a sexual being. This was not the first time a connection had been made between my pain and my sexuality. In fact, all of my caregivers had told me that, for many patients, there is a reason why the pain landed in the pelvic area. Issues about sex are often one of many factors contributing to pelvic pain. Iben said some of the women she'd treated for pelvic pain had a history of sexual trauma and others came from very sexually oppressed backgrounds. Physical sexual expression had been linked with shame and fear throughout my life, beginning in childhood.

When I was eleven years old, my unmarried, nineteen-year-old sister announced she was pregnant. That day, my dad looked at me and said, "You need to be one hundred percent good now."

Every time my mother would see someone kiss in public, she would always say, "That girl has no self-respect." The first time I kissed a boy was at age thirteen in my backyard during a game of truth or dare. I looked up to see my dad facing me in the window of the family room as he picked up his newspaper. Shame rocketed through my body like a wave of fire, and I couldn't sleep that night. I wrote my mother a long letter telling her to please call me in when it got dark because I wanted to be a good girl. Later that night, I crept into my parents' room and placed the letter by my mother's bedside. She never said a word about it. A few days later, I mustered up the courage to ask her whether she'd read the letter. "Yes," she said, and nothing more.

Twenty-six years later, I was standing at a grade-school reunion in Chicago when my first real crush (who had married a childhood classmate of mine) walked up to me. He started reminiscing about us at age sixteen, kissing in the backseat of a car all the way from a football game to my house while my girlfriend drove us home. He said I called him later, completely distraught and ashamed, vowing it would never happen again. I was especially embarrassed because my friend, the driver, was angry and judgmental about my unseemly behavior. At the reunion, my one-time teenage boyfriend said he had felt so sorry for me and had never forgotten it. I, on the other hand, had completely blocked it out, even though I have a great memory. Now, during this work with Iben, it occurred to me that this long-forgotten escapade had been the only time in my life that I'd been really passionate and not fully in control. I always dealt with the sexual part of myself through control and disengagement.

One December evening in 2010, right before my second bout with pelvic pain, I was having dinner with a few friends, and they realized that our mutual friend Jeff and I both had been raised Catholic. Someone mentioned that Catholicism had strict, controlling views about sexuality and wondered what that was like growing up. Jeff said no one really took those ideas to heart. I looked at him and said, "I did."

My views about sexuality had been changing throughout my journey toward body/mind/spirit wellness, and they no longer carried the huge moral overtones of my upbringing. I now considered sex to be a powerful, natural human expression that could be positive or negative, depending on the intention and circumstances. But now I realized I hadn't moved these ideas from my mind to my body.

After that epiphany, I consciously decided to let the sexual part of me live. As I sat in my backyard eating lunch one day, I closed my eyes and repeated, "I am a sexual being," several times. I said it quietly, just in case my neighbors were listening.

While I said my new mantra, "I am a sexual being," I saw the color red behind my closed eyes. I knew the area of my pelvic floor, the root chakra, was red in color, so this had meaning for me. Six months later, Iben mentioned in an unrelated conversation that the color red can also represent pain. Eventually, the connection between my sexuality and pain would reveal itself.

Pain and Anger

Right before I started working with Iben, I attended a yoga workshop. The instructor asked us to become mindful of our emotions as we held poses that stretched out the hip and pelvic area for what seemed like a decade. During the question-and-answer period, I mentioned that I didn't feel anything when I focused inward. Privately, I attributed this to my incredibly peaceful state and insight, so I was shocked at the instructor's response.

"This can be related to your past conditioning," she said. "What was it like in your home as a child?"

"Well, emotions weren't really allowed," I quickly replied.

Throughout my journey, different caregivers said or alluded that I never expressed anger. For example, at one of my early sessions with my psychologist, Jackie, she asked me, "Where is your anger?" Likewise, when I first met my physical therapist, Julie, she was amazed when I told her I never felt anger.

During the second flare-up of pain, Iben asked me to consider the last time I had expressed anger. I couldn't think of a single example! Then, Iben explained that the bladder often carries deep resentment and/or intense anger. Women get interstitial cystitis more often than men because society does not give women permission to show anger, so they hold it within their bodies.

I started to realize that the reason I didn't feel anger and resentment was because I'd become a master at quickly shoving those emotions inside. I also realized that this behavioral pattern had been entrenched during my childhood.

Suppressing Anger

My mother always told me that I'd been "really good" until I was about three years old, at which time I had developed a temper and would get angry when I had to go to bed. After I had children of my own, I thought, *Wait a minute! All three-year-olds buck the system!*

Perhaps that is why, whenever my mother read me the following poem (by Henry Wadsworth Longfellow), she would tell me it reminded her of me.

There was a little girl,
And she had a curl
Right in the center of her forehead.
When she was good
She was very, very good,
And when she was bad she was horrid.

In one of my first memories from about age four, I am sitting next to my mom in the car and she is scolding me for being such a "Crabby Appleton." I can remember sitting there quietly and steaming inside. Of all the negative emotions not allowed in my childhood home, anger was at the top of the list. So I'd learned at an early age to suppress it. Sometimes, I would cry and talk about my hurt or disappointment, but I stopped showing anger, especially in a physical way.

When I found and read my old journal, I realized that this pattern of shoving in my negative emotions had continued throughout my teens. The following passage was written at age eighteen:

> Hopefully, I can learn how to get my emotions out where they are felt, instead of bottling them up for home because my parents treat me with harsh words when I pour out my emotions on them. It's hard for them to understand that it isn't them; I'm just getting things out. I have to learn to stop fearing rejection and release how I feel when I'm feeling it. It will help people to see that I am human, and it will be healthy for me, too. I'll be more honest that way. It will take a lot of growing to achieve this end.

As a teenager, I encouraged myself to let out my emotions, but at the same time I knew that I didn't feel safe to express how I was truly feeling. I would continue this pattern for thirty more years, until pelvic pain stopped me in my tracks and I decided to heal. My eighteen-year-old self was right: It had taken a lot of growth before I felt secure enough to release my negative emotions.

Admitting It

One day, my sixteen-year-old son, without knowing about the emotional work I was doing, said, "Mom, you talk about being angry, but you never show it. You need to let it out."

Well, that second flare-up was really making me mad! After being pain-free for so long and doing so much work, I was livid about having to experience the pain again. So, when I picked up my son, Alex, at school the next day, I admitted for the first time that I was angry and even used a few expletives! Alex said he was actually relieved not to be the only one in the family feeling rage.

I asked, "Does knowing I'm in pain scare you?"

"Sometimes," he said.

"Is it weird to hear that I get angry?"

"No, Mom. I know you."

And he did. My son is one of the first people who truly saw me and accepted all sides of me. Ever since I held him on the day he was born, I have felt relaxed and safe with him. He is expressive and emotional, and in accepting and loving that part of him as his mother, I also accepted and loved that part of myself. It makes sense that he was the first person I felt safe enough with to express my anger.

Letting It Out

When my second bout of pelvic pain stretched into its fourth month, I was exhausted and upset. The relentless, nervy pain in my bladder weighed on me, and I was scared it would never subside. I was also really angry that the pain had returned after I'd worked so diligently for years to get past it. It felt like no matter how hard I tried, the goodness of life was being withheld from me.

One night when everyone was in bed, I started punching the couch cushions. Katherine came into the dark living room and asked in a dazed, sleepy tone, "Is everything okay?" I told her I was just getting out some frustration. She walked back to bed, probably thinking her mother was a little nuts.

The next day, I was sitting on the living room floor after doing some stretching, and thoughts of people and situations throughout my life that had ticked me off just kept appearing in my mind. Most of the memories were from preschool and grade school years, when I felt pushed into a subordinate role by other kids or my older siblings. Again, I punched those cushions to let out some pent-up anger. To my surprise, while I was beating up the couch, my clenched pelvic-floor muscles started to relax—the exact opposite of what I would have expected to happen! Strangely, it felt like I was clearing out space within me, letting go of what I no longer wanted to carry.

When my kids came home from school that day, they asked me about the pounding noises that had disturbed their sleep the night before. I told them that throughout my life I had never expressed my anger, and now it felt good to physically let out my frustration with the pain I was experiencing.

"That's a good thing for you, Mom," my son said.

Then, the three of us talked about how we express anger and what is productive and what isn't. There, in my own home and with my own children, I felt accepted. The angry, frustrated, discouraged me no longer had to hide to feel loved.

Finding More Release Valves

Iben encouraged me to let out my anger in physical ways so that energy wouldn't be held in my body. But it was really difficult for me to tap into and express my anger. I bought a punching bag, and the first thing I did was cover it with a flowery material so it matched the tablecloth on the back patio. A week later, I noticed it hanging out there and had to smile at the symbolism: I always covered up my anger so life would seem pretty. Expressing my anger in a physical way wasn't natural for me, and after those first two incidences, my couch never received another blow, and I still haven't punched that punching bag.

However, Iben knew that expressing my anger was crucial, so she used a lot of other avenues to help me release it. First, she had me write letters to the targets of my frustration, instructing me to pour out exactly how I was feeling without editing or holding back on the language. Those letters were never sent, but I did read every nasty word to Iben. While I was reading, several times she gave me a pillow and instructed me to place it over my face and scream into it to release some of the rage.

Next, as Iben placed her hands lightly on my fully clothed body, I told her about the people and experiences that had angered me. When she placed her hands gently over my bladder area, more anger and tears erupted. Lying there on Iben's table, talking about my anger with my nose running and my face wet with tears, I felt completely exposed. But when I looked up into Iben's face, her sparkly blue eyes reflected only intense love. Expressing my anger was scary for me, and receiving this unconditional acceptance felt very meaningful and healing.

Iben then asked me to rewrite each of my letters so that every sentence began with "I." This helped me to own my feelings and reactions, to take back my power, and to feel more in control and less like a victim.

Finally, Iben showed me how to go into lion's pose (yoga) and to vocally release some of the carried emotion. In this activity, I sat on my heels with my knees apart and reached forward to place my hands on the ground in front of my legs, bending forward at the waist and placing my forehead on the ground. After each deep breath, I moved into this position, stuck out my tongue and pointed it downward toward my chin and expelled air with a loud, deep, raspy tone. With each loud exhale, I imagined the energy/breath coming up from the pelvic-floor area, all the way up and out of my body.

One day as Alex was leaving on a trip, he made some cutting remarks that made me really mad. When he left and I was alone, I did the vocal release in the lion's pose. More and more emotion kept bubbling up, and it seemed to be coming forth physically, too. I felt a burning sensation in the center of my chest; I also gagged and spit up phlegm and saliva. After two hours, it felt like there was nothing left to get out, and I felt lighter, more peaceful, and pain-free.

A few weeks later, when my marital dynamics were annoying me and I was physically flared up again, Iben came to my house. She got in my face, knowing exactly what to say to spark my underlying rage. Good thing she had pillows to ward off the blows!

This was new territory for me, but I knew deep down that releasing this pent-up energy was crucial for my healing. Every time I released my anger, no matter the method, my nervous system would feel calmer and my pain levels would drop.

Iben encouraged me by saying, "Fear takes energy from you, but anger is a beautiful tool that can push your growth. Anger is a way to maintain boundaries and to say, "That's enough."

Developing Compassion

My acupuncturist, Pam, told me that sometimes we are alone on our journey. We have to go through things first; then, we have more to share with others.

I knew this was true from my past experiences. Before my bulging disc pressed on the nerve root in my neck, I'd had no idea how intense nerve pain could be. But after experiencing it myself, I could empathize with what my patients were going through.

When Katherine was born, I'd suffered seizures and a small stroke and landed in a neurological intensive care unit. A few years later, I'd walked into that same ICU as a physical therapist. I told a few patients that, although I had no idea how it felt to deal with the aftermath of a major stroke, I did know how it felt to wake up in that room, be pulled off a respirator, and hear about my seizures and stroke for the first time.

Even though helping others deal with pain and horrific disability had always been my job, living with pelvic pain has given me a whole new perspective. Now, when I see the old and infirm coping with their limitations, I no longer feel separate from them. I can picture myself carrying a similar burden, and I feel a stronger bond of shared humanity.

During my second flare-up of pelvic pain, I started to appreciate that, prior to my illness, my circle of compassion had not encompassed people with depression or chronic pain. I recalled that, right before my pain first began, when a woman in the gym's locker room told me about her battle with depression, I'd taken a step backward and made a mental note to avoid intense conversation with her in the future.

Other similar memories surfaced. For example, when I was a new therapist in the 1980s, a woman on a plane tried to talk with me about fibromyalgia. Although I'd tried to look interested, I had not really listened and thought she probably suffered from some psychological disorder that had created the condition. When other therapists would talk about treating patients with chronic pain, I'd think or even say out loud that I didn't know how they could do it. I also had no idea how therapists could work with someone with pelvic issues; I'd felt that those patients and their problems were somehow separate and a little beneath me.

After the pain, I thought it was curious, and perhaps not coincidental, that my illness had firmly planted me among the group of people I used to shun. I wondered whether the reason I'd been previously unable to accept others with those conditions was because I'd been shut off from these aspects of myself.

One painful day during the second flare-up of pelvic pain, I was sitting in the whirlpool at the gym. A twenty-year-old guy sat to my right, and I noticed he had a tattoo that looked like death itself on his arm.

"I feel just like your tattoo today," I said.

"I feel like it every day," he responded.

Then, he glanced cautiously at me, and I saw his dark brown eyes brimming with pain.

We talked for forty-five minutes about our experiences with physical and emotional pain.

As I stepped out of the spa, I said, "I hope that wasn't too much information."

He said I'd given him a lot to think about and thanked me.

After thanking him, too, I said, "It is really weird, but the last four times I've been in this whirlpool, I've met someone who shares at this deep level."

"That's no coincidence," he replied. "You opened up and you asked about my pain. We all have pain, but no one ever talks about it."

He was right. Before I developed chronic pelvic pain, I thought I was the only one who was hurting because many people suffer in silence or don't have an awareness of what they are carrying. Now, I realize that I am not alone and that suffering, just like joy, is an integral part of the human condition.

Later, I revealed to my friend Christine that I silently resented when others did not connect with me on an emotional level.

She commented, "Isn't that the same as your mom, only she silently resented when others *were* emotional?"

I had to smile, because in many ways, my mother and I are different sides of the same coin. Once I allowed myself to look at and accept all sides of me, even the not-so-pretty sides, I began to have compassion for myself, which actually enabled me to have more compassion for other people, too. I started to realize that most people were like me—unaware of their emotions, playing out the same old patterns, and just trying to survive it all.

Dealing with Imperfection

During the second bout with pelvic pain, I sometimes felt like I was falling into despair. My journal entry from October of 2011 shows this discouragement:

> I am embarrassed that I am still hurting, and I feel like I'm not doing something right. It feels like the pain is my fault. I feel like I'm supposed to get over this and I'm failing.

Soon after writing that, I found a passage in my journal written one year into my pain that gave me encouragement:

> I am not responsible for my life playing out a certain way. I don't have to perform or achieve my life. Illness and adversity are part of the human condition. I am human. I have not failed. I need to just get through the best I can. I have been forced to be quiet, and there is beauty in this, too.

My internal drive for physical and spiritual perfection and my frustration at not meeting the ideal often cropped up. Iben would always remind me that the goal was progress and not perfection. She would also say, "We are not here to be perfect; we are here to be awake." She encouraged me that I was still healing through the layers, and even though I was in a valley again, I was still moving forward.

Moving Down the Healing Path

I chose the title "Full Circle" for this chapter because it describes coming around again to the same painful experience—albeit, with a new perspective. However, in many ways the image of a circle doesn't capture my healing journey. The pain often pushed me to grow in self-awareness, and I know this process of self-discovery will continue throughout my life and I'll never have complete closure, like a circle. During the second bout of pain, I realized that every time the pain returned and pushed me, my insight would grow. So this journey could be depicted like a timeline, rather than a circle, with occasional high-frequency oscillations, and during these rough spots, the trajectory of the line ascends.

As I've told several friends, "This pain is like an intense learning course for my soul, and sometimes I wonder who put me on the roster or why I signed up for the course!"

I'm not one who responds to suffering with the stoicism of some pious saint. I get mad, discouraged, and sad. I sit in my living room crying in the dark. But then, support flows from within and from without, lifting me up and pushing me on down the healing path.

One Sunday while I sat in discomfort in church, the minister said, "You can be beaten down, only to get up and be beaten down again. But when you are down there, only you can stop your heart from lifting."

And I thought: *That was meant for me! This pain always pries my heart open a little more.*

11

Treating the
Body-Mind-Spirit

Over the years, several caregivers used the analogy of peeling layers off an onion to describe the healing process. I would agree and add that, also similar to peeling an onion, my healing was often accompanied by a lot of tears.

Looking back on this journey, it seems like different types of therapy were effective for healing different layers. For example, in the very beginning when the pain was intense, physical treatments helped calm my body and mind. Later, deep introspection with my life coach, Iben, helped me to shed many layers and arrive at a more peaceful place in my body and in my life. Then, during my second bout of pelvic pain, alternative treatments that simultaneously worked at the body, mind, and spirit helped me heal through more layers. In this chapter, I explore those alternative treatments from the perspective of both a patient and a therapist.

Voice Lessons as Therapy

Starting in the summer of 2011, I took a year of voice lessons from Cris, a petite Chinese man in his early thirties with a powerful, peaceful spirit and a voice almost as high as mine.

On our first lesson, when Cris didn't know about my condition yet, he observed, "If we can get your pelvic floor relaxed, then you are good to go."

During our sessions, he looked at my full posture and gave me cues to activate or relax different parts of my body, all with the aim of producing a clear, resonant tone. The way Cris analyzed the whole body was similar to how I'd once helped my patients who had suffered a stroke or brain injury. The only difference was the end motor skill: For Cris, it was the quality of my voice; for me, it was the patient's ability to sit, stand, and walk.

When his mentor, Karen Clark, was visiting the area, Cris encouraged me to have a lesson with her, saying she used the Feldenkrais approach even more than he did during his lessons. *Really? Feldenkrais?* I thought. That was the treatment approach my colleagues and I had completely discounted twenty years before when it was presented in a seminar. But now I couldn't deny that some Feldenkrais techniques had been very helpful in enhancing my voice, calming my body, and decreasing my pain. These techniques, which seemed to mirror how I naturally worked as a physical therapist, had snuck in through the back door.

To attain breath control while singing, the diaphragm contracts and descends and the pelvic-floor muscles relax. So the quality of my voice became another measure of the state of tension in this area. Singing also required me to relax the pelvic floor while expressing myself in a public way, which wasn't always easy.

After almost a year of lessons, Cris asked me to sing a short Mozart solo for a church memorial. I practiced for a month, until it sounded good in the shower, in the car, and even in front of the choir. But on the day of the service, my body tightened up and my voice sounded squeaky as it strained toward the high notes, all the dissonance blatantly magnified by the microphone.

As I sat in shock after the service, Cris and my friends approached me. They were honest but very kind, and they all encouraged me to keep singing so I could become more comfortable. When I expressed disappointment with myself, a friend told me to use my ego to push myself forward but never to slap myself in the face. Another choir mate told me to just take the word "failure" out of my vocabulary. When I came home and told my husband and son about the fiasco, they didn't care. My son hugged me and told me to not worry about it.

The people around me mirrored how I should treat myself. I guess I didn't need to be perfect in order to be loved, after all. I'd started singing lessons to develop a better voice for choir, but those lessons ended up being a powerful healing tool for my body, mind, and spirit.

Myofascial Release

Four years after my pain began, I received a brochure in the mail from the John Barnes' Myofascial Release Approach for a course titled Fascial Pelvis. The general term, myofascial release, has been used to describe many types of treatments that work on the connective tissue throughout the body. John Barnes has combined many of the principles of myofascial release with different perspectives to create a therapeutic approach referred to throughout this book as Myofascial Release.

Before my illness, I used to roll my eyes when these mailers came to my house. It had always bothered me that John Barnes was using his physical therapy degree as a credential because I didn't think the treatment was valid. But now I looked at the mailer with interest.

I remembered that, a few years earlier when Julie had first seen my spontaneous movements, she'd told me she had seen others move in a similar way when she took this Fascial Pelvis course, and the movements were called "unwinding." So I was curious about the course. In addition, I had to complete thirty hours of continuing education in the next few months to renew my physical therapy license, and I was still in a little discomfort for part of each day. The course seemed to meet my needs as both a patient and a therapist, so I signed up.

It had been a long time since I'd traveled alone and thirty years since I'd gone to a destination where no one knew me. So I was excited and a little nervous when I flew to Arizona in October of 2011, and drove up to a plateau in Sedona, where the motel and course were located.

That evening as I watched the sun set over the canyon, I struck up a conversation with two guys about my age. One of them was going to the same class as I, and it was the sixth course he had taken with John Barnes. When I told him about my spontaneous movements, he said participants had learned how to do self-unwinding movements in an advanced course of the series.

The next day before the class began, I walked over to John Barnes and introduced myself. I told him about my pain condition and about the spontaneous body movements I had experienced. He told me that spontaneous unwinding was rare, but it could happen. He reassured me that it was a natural part of healing and there was nothing wrong with me. He said that maybe the movements were continuing because I had not fully resolved what I had begun. He recommended that I attend a couple of sessions at his treatment center, Therapy on the Rocks, during the week I was taking the course.

The Theory

The foundation of the Myofascial Release approach is that we all have an inherent capability to heal ourselves and to aid each other in healing. John Barnes' theory is that past trauma—like surgery, physical injuries, and even unexpressed psychological trauma—can create restrictions in the fascia, which eventually can lead to abnormal stresses and ultimately to pain and dysfunction. Fascia is the collagenous (elastic) connective tissue that envelops all our internal structures, providing support and separation for the structures and decreasing the friction between them, which is necessary for movement.

In her book *Women's Bodies, Women's Wisdom*, Christiane Northrup, MD, describes fascia as a "crystalline matrix" that connects all parts of the body. She postulates that fascia may aid in the transmission of energy and information throughout the body. John Barnes described fascia in a similar way during his course. The idea that fascia may be related to energy flow in the body matched my personal experience. The spontaneous body movements I experience definitely stretch the fascia, and after those movements, I often feel a light tingling throughout my body that mimics the sensation I've experienced with other energy work, such as acupuncture and Reiki.

The Practice

During a Myofascial Release treatment, both the patient and the caregiver go into a quiet meditative state. The therapist then applies a prolonged gentle stretch to different tissues, with each stretch lasting three to five minutes. Applying tension to the fascia at one part of the body can affect remote body sites because the fascia throughout the body is all connected. It is postulated that with prolonged gentle stress, the elastic component of the fascia relaxes first, and then, over time, the gelatinous portion of the fascia becomes more fluid. It is this latter change that is considered to be most effective in producing permanent change in the tissues.

At the workshop, after each technique was demonstrated, we found a new partner and practiced that technique, with each person taking a turn in both the patient and the therapist role.

After John Barnes demonstrated the first technique, my partner lay on the treatment table while I applied a sustained, light stretch to the side of her torso. After a few minutes, her whole body started to stretch and move in random ways. I looked around the room and saw other people moving, too. Before my illness, I would have chalked up these observations to group hysteria or the power of suggestion. But without even knowing they existed, I had experienced similar movements when I was alone in my own home.

During the seminar, John talked about unwinding and introduced another type of healing movement, called rebounding, in which the body moves in a rapid oscillatory motion.

At the break, I bounded on stage and told him, "A few months after my body started to unwind on its own, it also began rebounding, like you just demonstrated. My body moves in one other way, too."

Then, I demonstrated how my entire body would bounce rapidly, which happened when I relaxed and allowed it to happen.

Smiling, John said, "That's jiggling."

I thought he was teasing, so I replied curtly, "Well, it's nice to have names for this stuff." Then, I turned and quickly left the stage.

Later, I found out John hadn't been joking and that jiggling really is the name he'd given to the third type of healing/releasing movement he demonstrates in his courses. The fact that all three movements happened to me before I had any knowledge of their existence and when I was alone in my own home helped validate this mind-body treatment for me.

Therapy on the Rocks

After the first long day of the Barnes course, I checked in for a Myofascial Release treatment at Therapy on the Rocks. I was escorted to a narrow treatment room on the second floor. I walked straight to the full-length window to look at the trees and the wide, running creek peacefully illuminated by the last light of day. Then, I stripped to my underwear and slipped under the sheet on the treatment table.

The practitioner knocked on the door, glided into the room, and introduced herself. Donna looked healthy and hearty, and she put me immediately at ease with her warm voice and gentle demeanor. She listened intently as I recounted my pelvic pain history. Then, she placed her hand across the six-inch scar from my two Cesarean sections. After a minute or so of light pressure, my body started to unwind. Sometimes, a posture would be sustained and my body would start to shake.

Donna continued the gentle pressure on my lower abdomen, and my tears began to rush out. Memories of being little, vulnerable, and alone flooded back, and I began to talk about them.

Donna asked me to describe the emotions those memories brought back, and as I did, anger suddenly rose up. I told Donna I was mad at my mother for not nurturing me and that I felt discounted and managed. Donna told me to be a little girl again and to tell my mother what I was feeling, which I did. Then, she instructed me to go into those scenes as an adult and to comfort and love the little me. All the while, Donna kept up the gentle pressure on my lower abdomen, until my memories subsided, my emotions calmed, and my body stopped moving.

Then, Donna slowly moved her hands to my left lower-pelvic area and pressed firmly on the scar from my hernia surgery. When she did this, a distant memory flooded back: I was sixteen and in a hospital room recovering from hernia surgery, and my mom was sitting across the room entertaining her friend. This theme—a lack of connection and tenderness from my mother, especially when I was hurting—ran through all the memories that surfaced during the session. Again, when the memories stopped, my body and emotions were calm.

At the end of the session, Donna told me to lie quietly for a few minutes before I got up and dressed. As she walked toward the door, she instructed me to be still and to listen to my inner voice for the message I was to come away with. In my mind, I immediately heard, *You are not alone*, and said out loud, "I have it!"

Donna turned at the doorway and smiled. "Take your time and wait for the message," she repeated. She closed the door quietly behind her, and I lay there alone in silence. After a few minutes, I suddenly felt a fullness in my heart; it felt like it was going to burst as another thought came through: *You are loved*. I knew that both of those messages were true.

Earlier that day during the workshop, I'd had a low level of bladder pain that had bothered me for a few hours, and my pelvic-floor muscles had been tight. After my session with Donna, I noticed that my discomfort was gone, and I remained pain-free for the remainder of the course.

The day after my session with Donna, I approached John Barnes during a break and told him I had attended therapy at his center the night before. I relayed that I was well-acquainted with the main issues in my life and had worked through many of them at the mind and energy level, so I was surprised that I seemed to be carrying this stuff deep within the structure of my body. He smiled and nodded. When I told him I'd felt a bit lightheaded and destabilized after my treatment, he reassured me it was a normal part of the process and actually a good sign.

Two days later, when I had barely recovered from my first treatment, it was time to return to Therapy on the Rocks. This time, Donna placed her hands on the muscles of my inner-upper thigh and asked me, "What is held in this part of your body?"

Instantly, memories of Katherine's traumatic birth flooded back. I'd endured twenty-four hours of labor, an emergency Cesarean section, double pneumonia, seizures, and a stroke. I was in a medically-induced coma and on a respirator for about a week, with my blood pressure soaring, even though I was on the most potent blood pressure medications available. What surfaced during my second therapy session with Donna was not the physical trauma, but rather, lots of anger. I was angry that my mother had taken over and my baby had bonded with her. I was angry that my mother had encouraged my husband to go to work and sent him and my dad to visit me at the hospital for only an hour each night. At the time, I didn't think it was right to have any needs of my own because everyone was pitching in to take care of my baby. But during that Myofascial Release session, I felt my suppressed anger and hurt that no one had been there to support me after such trauma.

Donna encouraged me to let out all these emotions, saying, "You don't have to be a good girl."

When a scream erupted, she smiled gently and said, "I knew you had it in you."

Donna warned me that kicking a pebble can often lead to an avalanche. She was right. That night, I woke up at about two in the morning, and for the next couple of hours, I felt rage. This was quite a new experience for me. Memories from a lifetime popped into my head, all related to my mom and my suppressed anger. I took Donna's advice and talked with my deceased mom, expressing all my pent-up feelings. I went into lion's pose, as Iben had showed me, and expelled loud raspy breaths into my pillow. Like before, I felt burning in my chest and gagging in my throat, and I coughed up phlegm and saliva. It was intense—and both awful and awe-full.

Back to Class

On the last day of the Barnes course, I felt really tired but also more open, relaxed, and authentically me.

One of the first techniques of the day was a very gentle neck pull (called traction), which was held for about five minutes. I took the patient role first, and a guy about my age cradled my head and pulled it lightly away from my body. Right away, I saw an image of my dad in his casket and me standing over him, alone and in shock. Next, I saw myself standing over my mother's casket with the same emotions washing over me. My partner quietly moved with me as my body unwound and I started to sob, my nose running and tears flowing down my face.

After about ten minutes, John Barnes asked the group to switch roles. With his hands still on my head, my partner said, "That was awesome." I told him about the images, and he encouraged me to open up and let in the love of my parents.

Letting Go of Old Beliefs

The week after I returned from Sedona, the healing seemed to continue. Every night I woke up at about two in the morning with my body spontaneously unwinding. To avoid disturbing Alex, I went into the living room and moved all over the floor out there. After about an hour, the movements would stop and I'd crawl back into bed. I wondered if I were just stirring up stuff and perhaps making my condition worse. But Dr. Ryan, Julie, and Iben all told me it was important to work through the emotions I was carrying at the body level. All of them also thought I would eventually land in a pain-free spot again.

One morning I woke up with a list of beliefs on my mind that I realized I had been carrying throughout my life:

- Tenderness and love are hard to get.
- I need to be perfect in order to be loved.
- Life is hard.
- My body is stiff, inflexible, and a problem.

It was especially clear to me that I had been frustrated with my body from as early as I could remember. I decided those beliefs no longer served me and I could let them go now.

That week I had a physical therapy appointment. Julie now had a private practice and employed other skilled therapists. On that day I worked with Nicole, with whom I'd worked with previously.

Nicole reminded me a lot of myself before my illness. She was sensitive to emotional issues and naturally intuitive in her treatment style, but at the same time, she was very analytical and focused on the body. The first time she'd seen my body unwinding during a treatment, she'd wondered out loud if it weren't some sort of pathology. When I'd told her about my experiences in the Myofascial Release course, she'd questioned whether I was just stirring up stuff and exacerbating my pain.

On this visit, while Nicole gently internally stretched my pelvic-floor muscles, I talked with her about the beliefs that had popped into my head earlier that week. As we talked, it hit me: On some level, I'd been thinking that when I consciously let go of my belief, my body would change into a more fluid form within a week. Then, when my body remained stiff and inflexible, I became impatient and frustrated.

I told Nicole, "I just figured out that I slipped right back into my old belief that my body is a problem."

She said, "I am feeling a huge release in your muscles right now."

Just then, I felt a light tingling sensation at the top of my head, and I was momentarily overwhelmed by emotions of love and gratitude. Tears welled up in my eyes and rolled down my cheeks. As those feelings washed over me, Nicole said my pelvic-floor muscles completely let go and the tension was gone. In those few minutes, I directly experienced a tangible connection between my body, mind, and spirit.

Nicole looked at me with huge eyes and said, "Wow, that was awesome!"

(Six months later, the structure of my body would suddenly change in a profound way.)

CranioSacral Therapy

Several months before my pain began, I was teaching a physical therapy course at Western University of Health Sciences. When I learned that the therapist who headed the physical therapy department treated patients using the CranioSacral therapy (CST) method developed by John Upledger, an osteopathic physician (DO), my respect for the department head immediately plummeted.

Nine months later, after the pain had descended and I'd stopped teaching, my physical therapist, Julie, performed a treatment that relaxed my body and calmed my nervous system. When I asked her what she'd just done, she said she'd recently learned the technique in a CranioSacral therapy seminar. Who knew?

I decided to attend a couple CST courses to check it out. So, one month after the Myofascial Release course, I attended my first CST course, and three months later, in February of 2012, I attended a second CST course.

The Theory

Originally developed in 1899, by William Sutherland, an osteopath, craniosacral therapy (also known as craniosacral bodywork) is the biodynamic manipulation of the connective tissue of the cranium (skull), spine, and the sacrum (the thick, triangular bone near the base of the spine). CST practitioners and advocates believe that immobilization of any part of the craniosacral system can result in illness, chronic pain, and dysfunction of the nerves surrounding the brain and spinal cord. With CST, the practitioner applies very light pressure to the skull and the spine, and these gentle motions are used to subtly alter the alignment of cranial and spinal bones as well as the underlying membranes and cerebrospinal fluid surrounding the brain and spinal cord. Therapists feel for restrictions and perform gentle tractions and techniques to restore optimal movement within the system.

Beginning in the 1970s, John Upledger, DO, developed his own method, referred to as CranioSacral therapy. With his approach, therapists feel the craniosacral rhythm, which is a distinctive, subtle, and body-wide motion. Dr. Upledger postulated that this delicate rhythm originates from the production and reabsorption of cerebrospinal fluid, which is then transmitted throughout the body via the fascia. His approach emphasizes that the vitality of this rhythm reflects the overall health of the person's central nervous system, or "life force." John Barnes postulates that this same rhythm reflects a person's electromagnetic energy, or "essence."

In the CranioSacral course, the instructors described what had happened to me in Sedona. As the body responds to the hands-on work, the patient's thoughts, feelings, and memories sometimes surface. A common phrase in CST circles is, "There can be issues in the tissues." This may be another example of cellular memory, the idea that experiences and belief systems can be stored not only in the brain but also throughout the body. In an adjunct treatment of CST called SomatoEmotional release, the therapist tracks subtle changes in the body (somatic), including craniosacral rhythm, to validate the patient's expressed thoughts, words, and feelings as they relate to the tissue releases.

CranioSacral therapy, Myofascial Release, and cellular memory reprogramming all emphasize that we have an innate ability to heal ourselves and to aid each other in healing. Even though some of the techniques and terminology are different, they all seem to tap into a similar mind-body phenomenon.

Before my pain, my mind would have closed as soon as the theory for each of these treatments was presented because these treatments are outside of mainstream medicine and there is little hard evidence to validate them. But now, I cannot deny that these methods have helped decrease my pain. I decided to not let my mind be the gatekeeper for possible knowledge and to use my body as a case study, focusing on what I felt with my hands as a therapist and with my body as a patient.

The Practice

The first CranioSacral course I took emphasized the use of light pressures to mobilize the fascia covering the brain and spinal cord. The second course presented familiar concepts, such as energy work, fascial release, and the idea that repressed emotion or trauma can cause physical dysfunction.

At the beginning of the first course, my partner, Audrey, and I practiced using a very light touch (about the weight of a nickel on the skin) to appreciate the craniosacral rhythm throughout the body. When I was trying to feel this subtle sensation on Audrey's body, I could feel something, but at first I wondered whether I was just making it up. But while we worked, Audrey reported what she was feeling in her body, and it almost always matched the light sensations I was picking up with my hands. Likewise, when Audrey treated me, her description of what she felt with her hands almost always matched what I felt in my body. At times, it seemed like my hands were moving in tremendous arcs of motion, but when I opened my eyes, my hands were still. One time it felt like I was pressing heavily into Audrey's neck, but when I opened my eyes, I saw a space between my fingers and her body; I wasn't even touching her!

When Audrey was treating me, I sometimes felt tingling throughout my body. Other times, my body would just unwind in response to her touch. Since unwinding movements hadn't been discussed yet, I had to reassure Audrey I was okay.

In the second course, we practiced feeling for subtle turbulence in the tissues, which is thought to reflect trapped energy. Two students and the teacher, independently and without consulting one another, all put their hands on the same spot on my body. I'm not sure what they were picking up, but they all found it in the same spot—and it wasn't one I would have chosen based on my past pathologies. When I placed my hands on the body of a classmate, I felt an area of increased turbulence in her mid-abdomen. When the teacher used that student as a demonstration for class the next day, she treated the exact same spot. In the course we were taught several ways to determine where to work, and often three or four methods would point to the same location on the body.

Using manual skills and the intuitive sense to pick up on trapped energy or fascial restrictions truly would have sounded ridiculous to me a few short years ago. It still sounds sort of crazy, but when I experienced it with my own body and felt it with my own hands, this information was able to permeate my filters. I started to appreciate that, even though I didn't know exactly how they were working, some of these mind-body techniques had powerful effects. Over time, my experiences as a patient and as a therapist provided me with more validation of the merits of this mind-body approach.

Practicing with Skeptics

After my first CranioSacral course, I tried using a very light touch, just an intention of movement, when I performed self-treatment for my pelvic-floor area. To my surprise, this light touch was even more effective than my traditional therapy pressures in decreasing muscular tension and trigger points in the pelvic-floor muscles.

Then, Kelly, Lee, Jeff, and several other friends hopped onto my treatment table to let me practice on them. I used light pressures on their fully clothed bodies, and their responses were powerful and positive. After Alex read several of their grateful e-mails, my analytical engineer husband decided to let me practice on him. Later, he told me he thought it wouldn't hurt my feelings if he didn't have a response, since I'd already received so much positive feedback. But after his first session, he told me he felt calmer on the inside, and for the first time in years, when he woke up in the middle of the night, he could go right back to sleep instead of reading for an hour.

"Maybe it's just the power of suggestion," I teased.

"I don't think so, because I didn't think it would work," he admitted.

During his second treatment, Alex fell asleep on the table, and as I worked, I could feel tapping in the tissues, which is considered to be a sign of release and self-healing. The next day, he came home from work with an incredulous look on his face. He told me that he felt more weight bearing through his feet, like they were gripping the ground, and he felt balanced and ready for action. It felt just like when he was playing basketball in his twenties and was having a really good day on the court. He also said things that usually riled him up at work hadn't even bothered him.

"When you've talked about being centered or grounded, I thought it was just an emotional thing, but I actually felt it in my body."

That night when I told Katherine about her dad's experience, she said, "Well, if Dad can feel it, it must be real!"

After this direct experience, Alex thought this work had some validity, even though it was not formally studied or fully understood. When we were walking one night he said, "It's like a washing machine. If you have problems with the electrical system, it can sometimes lead to mechanical problems. Maybe you're working on the electrical system."

Discovering New "Apps"

From the beginning of my second flare-up starting in February of 2011, I attended physical therapy once a week. During that time, my pain levels dropped drastically, and most of my days were pain-free. However, my pelvic-floor muscles were still tense, and the level of spasm often fluctuated. It was discouraging, but it also made sense because, during this time, I was actively uncovering and healing lots of suppressed emotional trauma. All my therapists told me that this processing was not easy on the body, but they thought it would eventually lead to a resolution of my condition rather than the characteristic, periodic flare-ups often seen with patients who have chronic pelvic pain.

Three months after completing my second CranioSacral course, I told my physical therapist Nicole as we were starting treatment that I sensed my body was tired of the invasive internal work. I asked if she could check my pelvic-floor tension and then work on the external areas of my body first.

She checked the tightness of my pelvic-floor muscles and reported that they were about a five on a scale of one to ten, with ten being the tightest. Then, she had me lay on my right side and started to lightly stretch my left torso. After a few minutes, my body started to unwind.

I laughed and said, "This is how my body has been unwinding lately. Can you keep doing your therapy while I move?"

"Sure, let's just go with it." she replied.

My trunk and neck were moving in unpredictable, gentle ways when I began to see purple and green colors behind my closed eyelids. After a few minutes, Nicole and I both heard and felt *pop, pop, pop* in my lower back, and Nicole said the whole area immediately felt soft as butter. We looked at each other with amazement.

"Let's check my pelvic floor now," I said.

The muscle tension was zero on a one-to-ten scale and normal.

Two months later, Nicole started working on my body with typical manual therapy techniques, but she said my body wasn't responding well. So she switched to the lighter pressures, and my body started to subtly change under her hands. Nicole said she felt a "buzzing" in my central pelvic area, so she put her hand over the spot. Then, she put her other hand in the same location but on my back, saying she just had a sense that she needed to counteract the top pressure.

I told her, "In the CranioSacral course, that 'buzzing' is considered to be trapped energy. We were taught the technique you are doing; it's called a pelvic diaphragm release."

"It's so weird. It feels like my hands are burning up," she said. After a few minutes, she added, "My hands are moving a little bit by themselves!"

"Don't worry. That happens to me, too, when I'm working on people."

She checked my pelvic-floor tension both before and after this "energy" work. Once again, without working on the area directly, the tension had drastically dropped.

Over the next six months, Nicole's ability to perceive subtle changes in my body and use this lighter input progressively increased. I still have some musculo-skeletal issues, so Nicole's ability to combine this type of energy work with standard therapy has been extremely helpful for my healing.

Nicole and I often laugh about sharing these strange experiences. Before my pain began, I never considered that there was more to the body than just the physical form, and I thought any treatments that claimed to tap into something beyond the physical structure were invalid. Nicole felt the same way, and when a short presentation on Reiki was given in physical therapy school, she was completely skeptical. But when she was picked to be the subject for demonstration and the Reiki practitioner put her hands on Nicole's head, she immediately felt a sense of well-being flow over her and saw multiple colors that were beyond vivid swirling behind her closed eyelids. Still, even though she'd had that experience many years earlier, she'd never thought about it again until we began working together.

I started to wonder whether we all have an inherent capability to perceive this "energy" and use our hands to help each other heal and some people have just tapped into it. One night when I was having dinner with my friend Carolyn, she brought along a colleague of hers who was a physician. When I told this doctor about my experiences, she said, "I like to compare the body to an iPhone. You and I may each have one, and they can do the same things. But now you've discovered a few more apps!"

12

Healing Old Wounds

In March of 2012, after my second CranioSacral course, my pain ramped up again, and I went to see Iben.

As usual, I tried to put a positive spin on my experience, saying, "There still are beautiful moments, and I think I'm still growing in awareness."

Iben called me out. "Pain is pain."

I started to cry and admitted, "I get so weary."

One day when my friend Lisa and I went for a walk, she confided that she never felt so alive than when she went through some intense, emotional family issues. She admitted that, even though she was grateful the trauma had passed, she missed experiencing her life with such intensity and clarity.

"I've been in that intense state for years now," I said. "And I've learned a lot. But I'm really, really ready for it to end."

Since I'd had positive experiences in my CranioSacral courses and I was in some discomfort, I decided to set up a few sessions with Karen Axelrod, the instructor of the course I'd just completed. During the first three months we worked together I experienced some surprising connections between my body, mind and spirit!

Shifting Structure

When I entered Karen's treatment room for the first time, I immediately noticed a familiar little statue of an angel cradling a tiny bird. On the day my mom died, my then nine-year-old daughter, Katherine, and I had gone to a Hallmark store, where this same statue had immediately caught our eyes. We knew we had to buy it as a remembrance of my mother, who loved birds and had exuded such peace in her waning years. Coincidently, one year after my mom died, her twin sister sent me the same statue and wrote that it reminded her of me. It made me smile to see that little angel peering down from Karen's shelf.

Karen asked what my intention was for the session.

"I want to feel safe in my body," I replied without hesitation. I went on to explain that when tensions arose in my home, I could sometimes feel my pelvic-floor muscles pull up tight. I wanted to be present in the situation without my body reacting in such a fearful way.

Karen moved her hands lightly around my body before settling on the front and back of my left-lower rib cage. Almost immediately, my calf muscles started cramping, pulling my feet downward and inward. Memories from throughout my life bubbled up, and they all had a common theme. In these recollections, I didn't feel safe to be myself and felt I had to "shrink to fit." As the memories surfaced, I also felt intense heartburn and my pelvic-floor muscles started to spasm.

"When did you stop feeling safe in your body?" Karen asked gently.

Behind my closed eyelids I saw three words written in red:

One

One

One

"I guess at age one," I said.

As the memories continued to surface, Karen asked me to focus on relaxing my calf and pelvic-floor muscles. After a time, she encouraged me to slowly move my ankles, bringing my feet into the position they would assume in standing. Then, she pressed on the bottoms of my feet.

"It's interesting," she commented. "Some of the kids I treat who don't feel safe emotionally actually walk on their toes."

That fit! My mother had often told me I didn't walk until I was eighteen months old, and then I just got up and started walking on my toes. Throughout my childhood I walked with my heels off the ground, and even as an adult my heels would occasionally raise up when I walked without shoes.

Later that evening, I was pondering why I'd stopped feeling safe in my body when I was a year old. Then, I remembered that I'd envisioned the word "one" three times and wondered if perhaps it referred to hour one, day one, and year one. That made sense, because when I was born, both my mother and I had almost died. Maybe the birth trauma had reset my nervous system to a higher level of activation and increased the tone of the muscles needed for the fight-or-flight response. The calves and buttocks are crucial for stability in running, and in my case, these muscles have always been tense and tight, even as a child and at rest.

I have had tight calf muscles, stiff ankles, and highly arched feet for my entire life. I even have a prominent bump where my calf muscles attach to the backs of my heels (calcaneous), because the bone remodeled itself in response to the constant pulling stress. When I was five, my parents took me to an orthopedic surgeon, who considered lengthening my calf tendons. Thankfully, I never underwent the surgery, but as an adult I attended physical therapy and performed stretching and soft-tissue work to correct this condition for years, with little change.

That evening after my session with Karen, my feet and ankles started to spontaneously move in the opposite direction of the way they'd been throughout my life. When I sat or stood with my feet flat on the ground, my lower leg gently moved forward and inward, my arches flattened, and my toes moved up and out, and this position would be maintained for several minutes. Like all of my spontaneous movements, I could stop the motion at any time. Yet, if I decided to allow it, the movement would continue without conscious effort.

Immediately, I began to analyze why this change was happening in my body. Perhaps childhood trauma had reset my nervous system at a higher state of activation, and now my brain got the message that the trauma was over. The muscles in my body that had always been ready to carry out the fight-or-flight response could now relax.

My body stayed in this relaxed posture for several weeks . . . until I became stressed, and then my old posture re-emerged. After that, my feet and ankles would switch between this relaxed mode and the older tense posture, depending on my experience at the time. Curiously, almost any time I've treated someone using these newfound energy techniques, my own feet and ankles spontaneously unwind and are very mobile at the end of the session.

Iben once explained that with fear we can become less present spiritually in our body and actually become less grounded. In some ways, walking on my toes is a perfect physical representation of not being present or grounded in my body.

These days, my calves and feet are often relaxed, and my toes often grip the ground. I frequently feel like my feet are firmly planted on the earth and literally feel more grounded, like I've finally decided to be fully present in my body.

Changing a posture and a pattern of a lifetime was surprising to me, and it demonstrated the connection between my body, mind, and spirit.

After my session with Karen, I also experienced major heartburn, which was something new to me. Dr. Ryan gave me an acid reducer. She reassured me that my heartburn was part of the healing process and not the start of a new condition. After two weeks, the discomfort subsided and has never returned.

Finally Feeling Grief

My next CranioSacral treatment was my father's show—filled with memories of times when I'd felt he didn't value me. At one point, I started to cry, and Karen asked me what was coming up.

"Right after my dad died, I was lying in bed in pain, and it felt like he was standing right next to me," I said. "I've never had that type of feeling before, but in my mind I heard him say, 'I'm sorry. I'm sorry. I didn't know.'"

When I'd initially sensed my dad's presence and again when I remembered the incident during my session with Karen, I didn't know it had a bigger context. Six months later, it would make more sense.

Meanwhile, at my CranioSacral session with Karen, she suggested I adopt my father's perspective and see myself through his eyes. Suddenly, there I was, once again with my parents, feeling generous, compassionate, and full of fear—and trying to control the situation. I saw myself reaching out to everyone around my dad but withholding from him. I was full of unexpressed anger that he didn't appreciate me and wasn't there for me. Seeing my part in our relationship helped me feel less like a victim and feel compassion for both my father and myself. My dad and I were both emotionally depleted and angry that the other person would not fill us up.

Tears bubbled up, and after a few minutes I said, "This is grief. I never cried for my dad, and I miss him."

Five years earlier, my father's decline had been the final emotional insult I'd tried to push in before my body rebelled with chronic pain. Now, I was ready to revisit his passing, feel my emotions, and let it go.

Speaking My Truth

In my next CranioSacral session, Karen put one hand on the front of my neck and the other hand on the back of my neck and cradled it for most of the session. When she did this, my neck felt really small, like a child's, and I had to trust her there.

Almost immediately, childhood memories of having my thoughts or feelings discounted as being untrue or selfish began to surface. I started to cry and said, "I had to hold myself tight because there was no room for error."

Still gently holding my neck, Karen observed, "There was no room for air."

The next week I found the letter I had written to my family almost five years earlier, informing them of my illness. In the middle of a full page of writing that brightly relayed all our family news was this paragraph:

Thank you for being so supportive about my medical issues at Dad's funeral. After having symptoms for a few months, I've finally been diagnosed with a chronic condition of the bladder called interstitial cystitis. It can be very painful and debilitating, but it can also be managed. It can go away, but it also tends to reoccur and flare up throughout your lifetime. They don't know what causes it, and there is no specific cure, but they do have ways to manage it. I'm on a few medications, and decreasing stress also helps. I've been feeling much better this past week—almost pain-free. I feel thankful that I have good, accessible, compassionate doctors, and Alex has been just wonderful.

When I'm feeling good, I have a newfound appreciation for even the smallest things in my life.

I thought I had clearly told my family about my illness, but this letter certainly didn't speak my truth. I was going through hell at the time, and I was very hurt and angry that no one had contacted me in the months following my father's death. I'd expected my family to pick up on my distress, and when they hadn't, I'd held my anger and resentment inside.

A few days later when I read this letter to Iben and told her about my session with Karen, she explained that I didn't feel safe being vulnerable. This is true. I didn't want to be seen as needy and demanding, which was a label I'd often received from my birth family. I realized that throughout my life, I often didn't feel safe enough to speak my inner truth.

Not So Unique

My daughter, Katherine, arrived home for spring break with a book from her college philosophy class, titled *The Wisdom of the Enneagram: The Complete Guide to Psychological and Spiritual Growth for the Nine Personality Types*, by Russ Hudson and Don Richard Riso. The enneagram is a psycho-spiritual typology that identifies and describes the unique characteristics of nine different human personality types. It is used to help people recognize and appreciate patterns of human behavior. Derived from several ancient spiritual traditions, the first "enneagon" of personality types was developed in the 1960s by Oscar Ichazo. Many variations of the "enneagram," as it is now commonly called, exist today; among the most widely recognized of these is the Riso-Hudson enneagram of personality types.

When I read the description of the type-two personality, "the helper," I was shocked at how closely it matched my experience. I wondered how these complete strangers could so closely describe my thought and behavioral patterns, pain, and healing path.

The basic desire of the type-two personality is to feel loved, and the basic fear is to be unloved or unwanted. During childhood, people with this personality type typically come to believe that love will not be simply given to them, and so they have to earn the affections of other people.

Within their families, they learn to be helpers, pleasers, and nurturers, and this pattern often extends to their other relationships. Even when other people acknowledge their kind actions, helpers often wonder whether other people would be as close to them if they weren't so generous and supportive. Although helpers often present an image of generosity and selflessness, they may actually have enormous expectations and unacknowledged emotional needs.

When helpers feel less lovable, they start to look for specific signs they are loved, and if another person expresses his or her love in a different way, it usually doesn't count. They might also try to mold others to meet their emotional needs.

The helper's loving self-image sometimes covers deep feelings of grief, anger, and resentment, and they work hard to repress or deny these feelings. If acknowledging their own needs was forbidden or seen as a form of selfishness in their childhood, type-twos further repress their needs, hurts, and self-doubt. Helpers are often unwilling to admit the severity of their own emptiness and suffering. If they continue to overextend themselves for others and to suppress their emotional needs or aggressive feelings, their health can suffer and they can develop physical symptoms of emotional problems (somatization disorders).

Helpers prefer to see themselves in the most positive light, so healing requires them to recognize their darker sides. They regain health when they learn to recognize and accept all of their feelings without censoring them and to instinctively respond to their own internal stress. By nature, helpers think that real love is scarce. When they rediscover there is within them an inner expression of divine love that cannot be conditioned, withheld, or diminished, it is liberating.

At the time I read Riso-Hudson's book, I had already come to the realization that the process of healing through the layers wasn't unique to me. Now, it seemed like the layers themselves weren't unique, either!

The next week I talked about my thoughts related to the enneagram with Iben, who had never read Riso-Hudson's book. She explained that we all want to get back to feeling a sense of unity and connection to God (the All One), and we often do this by trying to connect with each other. She said the enneagram seemed to describe how different people react to the fear of separation from God (the All One) and how they try to reconnect with others to alleviate this feeling.

When I read about my personality type, I could see two contrasting states: the fearful, constricting side of my nature and the connected, expanding side of my nature. I smiled in recognition of my expanding side and bristled when I saw my constricting side so clearly spelled out.

Iben encouraged me to be easy on myself. She explained that in this life, everything is filtered through the self, so no matter how aware I might become, I will never become an ethereal being who is above it all. Darn! She said I would always have a light side and a dark side as well as the potential to act from either place. Iben reminded me that awareness is not being perfect. Rather, it is knowing from which side I am coming at the moment and taking responsibility for how I think, feel, and behave in response.

Feeling My Fear

At my next appointment with Karen, she asked me what my intention was for that session.

"I want to look into my fear," I replied.

My rear end was tight, and I thought it had something to do with bracing at a subconscious level. Iben once told me that tightness in this part of the body is often related to fear or to feeling less-than. In his book *A Headache in the Pelvis*, Dr. David Wise proposes that pelvic-floor dysfunction often results from subconsciously contracting the gluteal muscles in response to stress. We all have areas where stress signals us, and the pelvic area is mine. In fact, I probably come from a long line of butt-squeezers! My father developed bursitis of his hips when he was stressed out, most likely from clenching all the gluteal muscles that attach there.

Karen asked me to feel the emotions related to the tightness in my posterior and then to slowly move in from the edges. When I did this, I felt a crinkling in my brain, which gradually expanded and strengthened.

"It feels like an electrical storm is going on in my brain." I observed.

As the sensation intensified, I groaned softly and moved into a fetal position, and then I started to shake all over. Karen wrapped her arms around me in support. After a few minutes, my brain and body became completely calm.

Karen explained that when animals are attacked, they often assume a fetal position to protect their vital organs. When the threat has passed, they shake all over to relieve the stress. These primitive responses matched what happened in my body.

"Now that you've experienced the fear physically, what do you think it's about?" Karen asked.

Immediately, the words popped out: "If I stay symptomatic, I can stay safe in my home."

Really? I thought, incredulously. *Do I really believe that, deep down?* I'd always considered myself to be positive and proactive, so it was strange to realize my subconscious might have a different agenda.

The next day I had a dream about taking off in the family car by myself without telling anyone. After three hours of driving, I ended up in a strange and remote area and couldn't find my way back home. Alex showed up for a brief time to help me navigate, but most of the time I was on my own. I drove into a lake, down train tracks, and finally jumped out of my car as it slid down a mountainside. I was never harmed, but I sure was out of control! I was even stopped by the police for having bald tires, which seemed to represent a lack of grounding and preparation on my part. It was clear to me that, on some level, I was unsure about my capability to move out into the world and afraid of stepping fully into my life.

Two days later, a woman from my spiritual group came up to me and announced, "Guess what our next topic is going to be?" She didn't wait for me to answer. "It's about fear."

I just smiled and thought, *Of course it is!*

Getting the Message

During my next session with Karen, I had a clear feeling that the right side of my pelvic area was working hard and the left side was an open space, a vacuum. This had particular meaning for me. Iben once told me that the right side of the body (primarily activated by the left hemisphere of the brain) represents the masculine, linear-thinking side of being and the left side of the body (primarily activated by the right hemisphere) represents the feminine, intuitive, creative side of being. Using this metaphor, one could say that before my illness I'd lived and breathed on the right side of my body and the left side was completely shut down. Maybe it wasn't a coincidence that every one of my physical issues (the stroke, neck injuries, back injury, major pelvic-floor spasm, and plantar fasciitis) occurred on my left side. Sometimes, metaphors do mirror real life!

As I lay on Karen's table feeling this imbalance, I thought about having worked so hard to be seen and loved, all the while hiding the truth of my basic nature. With this awareness, a light tingling poured into my left side, filling it up. Both sides of my pelvis felt the same for a few minutes . . . until Karen and I started talking about my career plans. Then, the right side started working hard again and the left side checked out. This clearly represented what was happening in my life. I was about ready to publish this book and start a business related to alternative healing when I thought I should get more training in orthopedics (the pinnacle of left-brained stuff) so I could be "useful."

Then and there, on Karen's treatment table, I realized it was time to be fully myself out in the world. Over the next week, validation poured in. Several people, including Iben and Julie, asked me to do energy work with them, and each session felt healing for both me and the person on the table. A friend of mine is learning Vedic astrology, and when she reviewed the chart related to my birth year, day, and hour, she told me I should do alternative healing, writing, and speaking and that I was very intuitive and creative by nature.

I also had a dream. It was a twist on a recurring dream of mine. At age thirty, I'd left my first job working full-time with brain-injured patients because I had suffered a cervical disc injury, and lifting patients often flared up my neck pain. For twenty years, I'd often dreamed of returning to this original job and my body continually letting me down. The week after my treatment with Karen, I again dreamed of going back to my old job, but this time it was to say goodbye. On my way out of the clinic, I passed a donation pile that contained some of my old clothing. I took a pair of jeans and said, "Oh, these are still my size." For me, this dream represented the fact that I was moving on but keeping some old skills that still fit.

I considered all these experiences to be signposts showing that I was on the right path. Since the beginning of my illness, specific words, books, and experiences had often popped up to clearly point the way out of the dark. Then, my pelvic floor started to tighten or relax in response to situations, giving me clear messages from my very core.

All of this is still happening, and recently the avenues for information have been expanding. Now, my dreams are often so clear that they are almost devoid of imagery, and when I am working with Karen, memories, mental images, and body sensations also speak my truth. Either I've removed quite a bit of static so the signals come through clearer, or I'm so dense that God/The Universe has to shout to keep me on track! It's probably a little bit of both.

13

Hope from the Holistic Perspective

In the spring of 2012, I was pain-free most of the time, but on a few occasions my bladder pain rose up to challenge me again. During this time, many insights gave me hope, and I learned about the nature of pain from my current vantage point.

The Body as a Reflection

When my pelvic pain first started, I found that researching the condition online escalated my anxiety and pain. So, early on, I decided to stop reading and to trust my competent caregivers, instead. But when I started sharing my healing experience with people who suffer from chronic pelvic pain, I decided to go online to update myself on any new or useful medical information about the condition.

I started by reading the Wikipedia page titled, "chronic prostatitis/ chronic pelvic pain syndrome," and to my surprise, some of the proposed theories for the condition matched what I had experienced in my own body over the past five years. Even though the literature used to support these claims was sparse, it was interesting how accurately this description paralleled my case.

The Wikipedia write-up proposed that chronic pelvic pain might result from a dysfunction in the neuro-endocrine system, which helps regulate the body's response to stress. There may also be a dysregulation of the nervous system at the local level causing myofascial pain and neurogenic inflammation, whereby nerve cells release substances that promote inflammation in the tissues. It is possible that an anxious disposition and chronic, unconscious tensing of the pelvic-floor muscles may lead to overstimulation of the pelvic nerves, which can lead to bladder pain.

This description of possible pathology matched my symptoms. Over the years, I've come to appreciate that my nervous system had probably been in a heightened state of activity long before my pain began, and I seemed to persistently tense my pelvic-floor muscles.

These responses in my body also reflected my psychological state. Through the process of trying to identify what caused and contributed to my pain, I realized I'd always held feelings of deep insecurity and was always looking for signs that I was loved. I learned I'd adopted these beliefs and behavior patterns in response to the traumas in my life and that this hyper-vigilant state of my body-mind had probably started very young and continued throughout my lifetime.

It makes sense that the parts of my body that would be involved in this prolonged and habitual response to stress would be tired and calling for my attention!

The Fear Factor

I didn't get far in my research, because right after I read the description of possible pathology in Wikipedia, my nervous system ramped up, my pelvic-floor muscles tightened, and my bladder hurt. For about two weeks, I felt intermittent discomfort in my bladder area, and the tension in my pelvic floor rose from a level one to a level five (on a scale of one to ten). Even after all my experiences of the body/mind/spirit connection, I quickly adopted this pathology description as my whole truth and thought of myself as broken.

When I arrived for my next physical therapy appointment with Nicole, I said, "Wow, this condition is really bad! If the part of my nervous system that responds to stress is having problems, then my fear of the condition is actually helping to create it. No wonder this condition is so hard deal with; there is a direct feedback loop between pain and fear."

It took me about a week to figure out that if the pain were related to fear, I could do something about it. I was sitting in church for the Sunday service, and my bladder was in a spasm and tender. Then, halfway through the service, I decided to consciously flow love to my bladder area. The pain completely stopped, and I was pain-free the entire day.

The next day, I was sitting in the passenger seat while my husband drove us to a show, and my bladder started hurting again. During the hour-long drive, I placed my hands over my lower abdomen and breathed deeply, gazing at all the trees on the side of the freeway, which at the time seemed oddly connected to me and comforting. My bladder pain completely subsided and did not return for days.

After about a week of these calming activities, I returned to a pain-free state again.

Iben told me that my experience was common among her clients who had chronic conditions. When clients heard medical information or labels about their condition, they often responded with fear, and this fear would create a stress reaction in their bodies, which then exacerbated the condition or maybe even helped to create it.

Over these healing years, I have let go of many fears and past emotional traumas. Now, I discovered that one of my biggest past traumas and fear triggers was the pain condition itself.

To deal with this, I decided that if/when my painful condition made another appearance, I would try to limit my fearful reaction. I would consciously calm my mind and treat myself with love and compassion. Iben also encouraged me to be gentle with myself when I was in pain and to ask myself, *What is the most self-loving thought, emotion, or action I can choose at this moment?*

The Reactive Body

Before my illness, I viewed my body as a machine that would occasionally break down in unpredictable ways and my doctor as a mechanic who I hoped could fix the problem.

Recently, my friend Bob commented that trees, animals, and all of nature were constantly responding to what was going on internally and externally, and it was no different for humans. I had to agree. Today, I see my body as a living, adaptive organism. This perspective always gives me hope, because if the body is reactive and malleable, change and healing are possible.

Several years ago, Iben explained that the body is the physical representation of the spirit on this earth. She said each of us is made up of different vibrational energies—which, in order of highest to lowest frequency, are spirit, thought, emotion, and the physical body. She explained that energy/information often flows from higher levels of vibration to lower levels. Thoughts are neutral, and it is our emotional reactions to thoughts that create reactions in the body.

I didn't need to adopt this idea of vibrational energy to appreciate that my emotional responses could easily change the physiology of my body. Through the process of uncovering, understanding, and moving through much of my past emotional trauma, my body changed: My calves relaxed and my ankles started to move; my buttocks and pelvic floor relaxed; my posture changed; and my pain levels dropped. In my experience, becoming aware of my emotional and behavioral patterns and altering them in positive directions directly influenced the unconscious, automatic reactions in my body.

Healing Takes Time

During my second bout of pain, I was really discouraged when the pain came back because I had worked so hard to move past it.

At this time, Iben encouraged me to be patient. She explained, "Your body has been changing for four years now, but you have lived with your old pattern for forty-six years. You have been changing for less than ten percent of the time that the pattern has been established. You have been working hard at the thought and emotion level, and it takes time for the body to catch up."

I also remembered what Dr. Ryan had told me five months into my pain. "You may be able to fix things mentally, but healing emotionally and physically takes time."

The fact that it takes time to change patterns in the body wasn't new to me; I saw it often when I was working with patients who had suffered damage to their nervous system. After a stroke or brain injury, many patients could move their body in only a few ways, and often these movement patterns weren't functional. I helped them relearn how to use their neuromuscular system differently, so they could move in more variable and functional ways. It was encouraging that, even after major damage to the nervous system, many patients learned to move differently. But they often reverted to their habitual patterns, especially when they were stressed. It took lots of time and practice before the new ways of moving became consistent and automatic.

When my pain reoccurred, I remembered these experiences and gave myself the following encouragement: *Be patient. You have learned new ways of activating your mind/body, but it takes lots of repetition before the system moves it from a novelty to a habit.*

Decoupling the Response

When memories and emotions surfaced during my CranioSacral sessions, sometimes my body automatically went into a stress response, which was similar every time. My calf muscles contracted, causing my feet to point downward; my buttocks and pelvic floor tightened; and my eyes squinted shut. Sometimes, I felt pain in my bladder or a crinkling sensation at the base of my brain. I suspect this had been my body's subtle response to stress for much of my life, and it became exaggerated and dominant during my years of pelvic pain.

In therapy, Iben and Karen (my CranioSacral therapist) helped me become more aware of my underlying emotions. They also calmed my automatic body reactions using energetic body work.

During my CranioSacral sessions, when memories/emotions surfaced and my body responded in its habitual way, Karen often encouraged me to completely relax my body while still feeling the emotions. By doing this, I was trying to break the strong link in my nervous system between my turbulent emotions/past trauma and the automatic stress response in my body. To see whether this process had been effective, Karen and Iben would occasionally ask me to mentally conjure up the emotional trigger while they monitored my body's response. Over time, I could envision many past traumas, and my body would remain relaxed.

Through my introspective work, many of my emotional triggers have dissipated, and now when I'm stressed, I don't automatically go into my habitual mind-body pattern. However, the tension in my body occasionally returns. This pattern is well established, and my body remembers. But once it is activated, it takes significantly less time and effort to curtail this response.

Pain and Suffering Are Different

During my second bout of pelvic pain when I was falling into despair, Iben told me the following story to encourage me: A very holy monk fell and hurt his knee. While he was sitting and holding his bleeding leg, another person on the path recognized him and wondered how he could be in pain when he was so spiritually advanced. The monk said, "As long as I have a body, I will have pain. I may have pain, but I do not suffer."

This concept made sense to me, because during my second bout of pain, I had grown a lot internally, and my suffering was significantly less than the first time around. Every time the pain has returned, I have more internal resources and even less suffering. Growing emotionally and spiritually has changed how I experience my painful condition.

This journey has been life-changing and simply awesome. But it has also been painful and difficult, and there were times when I felt like I was falling into despair. When that happened, my new perspectives about the relationship between the body/mind/spirit reassured me that I was on a healing path. All of these experiences increased my appreciation for the responsive, healing capability of the body/mind/spirit and gave me hope. For me, hope enhances the healing potential in my body.

$$\sim\!\!\mathfrak{O} \quad 14 \quad \mathfrak{O}\!\!\sim$$

Finding the Root

In February of 2012, as part of a woman's discussion group I was asked to share memories of the nicest things someone had done for me in my life. I chose to read a description of my relationship with Father John to the group, which I had written about a year before my pain began:

I arrived six weeks premature, and my mother hemorrhaged and almost died during my birth. One night, my parents called Father John to tell him that the doctors were worried that I wasn't going to survive until the morning. He drove over to bless me in the hospital, and later he baptized me in a formal ceremony.

We moved away when I was just six months old, but I would always remember his visits. My first memories are of him throwing me into the air and carrying me around on his shoulders. When I was about four, I remember asking my mother in the kitchen, "Do priests wear pajamas?" He bounded toward the kitchen in his bright, multicolored flannel pajamas, his booming voice echoing down the hall, "Do priests wear pajamas?" He was a big man, about 6' 4", with a deep, resonant voice and incredible passion.

When I was about six, he suggested that we walk with my parents to the park near our house in the dark of night. I have no memories of my parents ever playing with me at the park, but I do remember that night and Father John playing on the equipment with me.

When I was nine, Father John gave me a petosky stone that he'd found on the shores of his Lake Michigan home. It was actually a fossil, a group of cellular animals forever huddled together. He said, "We are all together and connected." Then he told me, "I'm your spiritual father."

When I was an adult, he wrote a recommendation for me to get into college and made the long trip to perform my marriage ceremony. He visited me in California, bringing unicorns for my four-year-old daughter and dinosaurs for my two-year-old son. He brought along a kite and taught my daughter how to fly it. It was the last day I was to see him, and it was magical.

Four months later, in June of 2012, I attended a CranioSacral appointment with Karen. I thought it was probably our last visit because I was feeling so good. In fact, I was planning to send this book to the editor that very day.

For about a half hour I lay on the table, feeling relaxed and with light tingling sensations throughout my body. A picture of my childhood bedroom came into my mind twice. Each time, I ignored it. The third time the image appeared, I said, "I don't know; I don't know. Something happened. Father John was there."

Karen asked me how old I was, and I knew I was four. This memory wasn't the practiced kind, where I see myself from the outside and it plays like a movie. It was from the perspective of me as a young child, and my body felt like it was right there.

When I got very quiet, Karen asked a few questions, such as, "Where are you in the room?" "What is your position?" and "What does your body feel like?"

Each answer was always very clear to me as the scene unfolded in my mind and in my body. I had a clear memory of being sexually molested at age four by Father John, my childhood hero.

Then, my bladder started to spasm and hurt, and Karen asked me what I was feeling.

"I'm so mad I want to sit my four-year-old self on his chest and just punch him over and over in the face."

Karen told me that was an option. So I punched into the air until my arms were tired.

Our session was almost over when she asked me what I needed her to do to aid my healing.

"I need you to put your hands on my throat because I wasn't able to talk about it," I said. "He told me I had to keep our secret."

As I left my session with Karen, I said, "This is so dramatic. It makes a great story. Too bad it's my life."

Questioning the Memory

My long-suppressed memory of Father John was so opposite to the story of my life, I wondered whether it was true. I had no evidence that it had happened, and I couldn't confront Father John because he'd died of a heart attack in the middle of an airport in Paris, France, twelve years earlier.

Then, I remembered something Iben often said. "The mind has prior conditioning and can deceive you, but the body doesn't lie."

I couldn't deny that my body had given me incredibly clear signals during my session with Karen. During the treatment, she told me she'd felt a huge knot of energy directly over my bladder. The day before, Nicole had told me she felt a lot of turbulence in that same area.

The following morning, I cried, shook, and unwound in Alex's arms, and I cried off and on throughout the day for much of that week. I felt just like I had after my mother died: grief, exhaustion, and relief. I thought, *Something must have happened because this reaction sure is real!*

The day after my memories surfaced with Karen, I had an appointment with Dr. Ryan, my family doctor and internist. When I told her about the memories of abuse, she told me she was sure it was true. She repeated what she'd told me in the early years of my pain: Things happen when we are little, and we bottle them up to keep surviving. But to fully heal, it has to come out. She added, "At this point, you are well aware of your emotions and reactions, and now you know how it all began."

She was right. Over the past five years, I came to realize that I had shut down much of the emotional, feminine, spiritual, and sexual sides of me, and I had been working hard to reawaken these aspects of myself. Now, I had an idea why I had shut down in the first place.

This memory was hard to accept, even after Dr. Ryan's validation. So, after my appointment, I sat in my car and called my brother. After hearing my story, he told me that he knew the memory was true. He'd gotten a bad sexual-type vibe from Father John when he'd gone camping with him as a young kid, and he'd never trusted him after that. He reminded me that he'd spent a lot of time with me when I was little (he was nine years older than me), and looking back, he remembered noticing a change in me at about age four.

I said, "Did you know Father John's last assignment in the church was to manage the pedophiles in his diocese? He was in charge of moving them into jobs and living quarters where they were less likely to be around children. He told Mom that sometimes it was difficult when they re-offended, but that even pedophiles deserve love."

The Story Beneath the Story

Although the memory of Father John's abuse was difficult to believe, it matched my life patterns. Now, I understood why I'd carried so much anger toward my mother and why I'd cataloged all the childhood memories in which I'd felt vulnerable and abandoned by her. It was clear why I remembered in detail every comment my parents made about sexual expression and why I had my first bout of cystitis in my twenties, when I had sexual intercourse for the first time. It also made sense why I thought I needed to be perfect in order to be safe and loved. These are just a few examples of the missing pieces of my puzzle that were filled in after the memory surfaced and I'd processed it.

Once I knew this ugly truth, many of my past experiences and thoughts made complete sense to me. I have often heard that when a person dies, all will be revealed to them. When I became aware of this memory, I felt like I'd died early and was let in on the story *beneath* my life story.

The morning after the memories surfaced, Alex and I talked about the deep, far-reaching impact of that horrific childhood experience.

"Everything is so complicated," Alex commented. "There are lots of layers, and things seem to be connected in ways we don't even know about."

"It's a bit like being in the *Wizard of Oz* and deciding to peek behind the curtain," I said.

"Yeah. And why would anyone want to do that?" he asked.

"To stop suffering."

Getting Guidance

Later that week, I made an appointment with my life coach, Iben. We had worked together on a weekly basis for a full year in 2010, and then sporadically, as needed. The process of unfolding and healing through the layers was ever continuing, and over the years, when I hit difficult layers I would call upon Iben for guidance. This new layer relating to Father John felt like major granite, so I called on Iben to help me through it. We met on a weekly basis for about four months, working to uncover, process, and heal my repressed sexual abuse.

In yet another example of serendipity, Iben had previously moved through her own sexual trauma. When she was in her twenties, she'd remembered being raped at age twelve and then witnessing a younger family member being abused in the same way. Over the past twenty years, she has helped a multitude of people work through experiences of sexual abuse.

I asked Iben, "How could I not remember the most crucial event of my life?"

She told me many children who suffer from sexual abuse suppress the trauma. When I expressed regret that I had kept this secret buried for so long and let it affect my life, Iben reminded me that I was only four when it happened. I couldn't expect myself to understand more than what I had learned intellectually up to that point. She told me that when this happened, in 1966, there was no concept that priests could be molesters, there was no box for this information, and I might not have been believed.

Unique Healing Paths

That week I called Jackie, the psychologist I had worked with during my first year and a half of pain. I was finishing this book and wanted to make sure the details I had written about her were true. While we were talking, I told her about the molestation memory that had recently surfaced.

She replied, "That was buried really deep."

"Do you think it's true?"

"Absolutely."

She told me that repressed sexual abuse was a huge thing to uncover and asked if I had help dealing with it. She wasn't convinced that seeing Iben and Karen was enough. My friend Christine, too, suggested I see a psychologist who specializes in sexual trauma, and another friend recommended I join a support group for people who have been sexually abused. None of those options resonated with me.

Dr. Ryan assured me that I was on a healing path and encouraged me to continue my current therapies. She said that Jackie had not seen me in over three years and had no idea of my growth over that time. She said that because of the work I had already done, uncovering this abuse now was a completely different experience than it would have been had I been hit with it several years ago. She said that working at the mind/body/spirit level all at once was a good fit for me.

She was right. For the first forty-five years of my life, I had ignored my body and spirit and lived only in my mind. But now I had developed new ways of living and knowing, and this capability had to be honored.

Through these experiences I began to appreciate that everyone has an individual response to trauma and a unique way to heal from it. Iben told me that the same act can have completely different impressions on a person, depending on the circumstances and who they are. She encouraged me to not directly compare my experiences with others and to honor my own healing process.

Levels of Awareness

A couple experiences made me wonder whether I had always carried the knowledge of Father John's abuse at a subconscious level in my mind and body.

Three months before the sexual-abuse memories surfaced, I attended a session of my women's group in which I was asked to share a few poems. Since I rarely read for pleasure, I didn't know what to bring. Then, I remembered I had written several poems for a class in college, and I found them tucked in the pages of my teenage journal. I distinctly remember writing these poems close to midnight when the library was about to close and all my other homework was done.

My poetry always poured onto the page with little conscious thought. When I wrote the following poem, I had no idea what it was about, but when I read it in March of 2012, I knew it was an expression of my suppressed rage. Then, when I uncovered the sexual assault a few months later, I understood the reason for this intense emotion.

It is wounded
Quick, slam the door and secure the bolt
Upon the anger steaming, the hurt screaming, the blood streaming
Keep the door polished
No one will know

It is seeping
Wipe the oozing from under the door
Pouring the anger steaming, the hurt screaming, the blood streaming
The careless arrows announce
Secretly tiring smiles tell
It is hidden

Expose the mind's own conspiracy
Locking the anger steaming, the hurt screaming, the blood streaming
Imprisoned stench reveals decaying horror
It is dead

An experience from my Hawaiian vacation in the summer of 2010 also pointed to a subconscious knowledge of the abuse. I was staying in a condo nestled in lush foliage and just steps from a private beach on the north side of Kauai.

On the first night in this peaceful, idyllic setting, I had a violent nightmare. In the dream, I was in a concentration camp, dressed in gray, and with my head shaved. I stood at the end of a long line in front of a table that held stacks of folded clothes. A rumor passed through the line that a beloved, blond-haired boy had been killed; everyone was in shock. We were instructed to gather our clothing in a certain order, and I was worried because I hadn't paid attention to the instructions. On the other side of the table was a big, glistening pool that had a menacing shark gliding through its waters. I knew that the penalty for a misstep was to be thrown into the pool. After selecting the wrong clothes, I was tossed into the pool, and the little boy thought to be dead immediately rose up out of the water.

The dream switched to a second scene. I was hiding other people from a black panther that was on the loose. Someone approached us with a dead carcass and assured us we were safe. The animal wasn't inherently dangerous, but sadly, someone had poisoned him to change his basic nature.

I woke up wondering why I'd had such a vivid, movie-like dream when I was feeling so peaceful. After thinking about the first part of the dream, I realized that it represented my internal life before I'd experienced all this personal growth. I was the young boy who was initially killed as well as the trapped, anxious woman trying to follow the rules and worrying about the predator. When the woman died, the child came alive again.

That afternoon in Hawaii, I remembered a conversation I'd had with my acupuncturist several years before. She told me that Native Americans gave significance to different animals and that some animals were "totems" or "guides" that represented certain meanings relating to a tribe, family, or person. So I went online and looked up the panther, and found this description by Ina Woolcott:

> *"Black Panther's Power includes astral travel, guardian energy, symbol of the feminine, death, and rebirth . . . reclaiming Power . . . They represent the life and power of the night. They can show us how to welcome the darkness and rouse the light within it. . . . The hairs that cover their lithe bodies, especially on the face, pick up subtle vibrations. This is symbolic for those with this guide. It is an indication of a need to pay attention to their feelings and honor the messages those feelings transmit. . . . Touch can be a significant path to explore to awaken ones concealed gifts. The black panther's sleek, smooth, and sensual coat has been linked to sexuality. If a panther comes into your life, it may be asking you to resolve old sexual issues or to embrace your sexuality fully."*

Body Intelligence

During my first visit with Iben after the abuse memories surfaced, we talked for about an hour, and then I lay fully clothed on her treatment table. She placed her hands over my bladder and said, "Oh, your poor bladder! It feels so raw and tender." That's exactly how it felt to me, too.

Iben explained, "This is a flare-up of cellular memory related to the sexual abuse. You don't feel safe. Your feelings of fear and pain were confronted with the idea that Father John was a good man and you had no right to doubt him. This cellular memory is the emotional and physical imprint on your body of how that felt."

The idea of cellular memory was not new to me. Over the years, Iben had often said that different parts of the body characteristically held different beliefs and imprints. Pelvic-floor tension is often related to fear of attack, feeling inferior, and not feeling safe to be your authentic self. Bladder pain is often linked with intense anger and resentment. Six months earlier during a Reiki seminar, Iben mentioned that bladder pain can also be related to a lack of emotional connection with the father.

Before my pain descended, I would have completely disregarded the idea of cellular memory. It still sounds simplistic and suspect that certain body areas carry specific beliefs and imprints. But now, I can't deny that the location of my physical symptoms directly matched the emotional and spiritual issues I carried.

My friend Bob, now eighty-nine years old, made the connection right away when I told him about the sexual abuse. He listened intently and then exclaimed, "That is so interesting. Your physical pain was in the same exact place as your emotional pain. When you started to relax on the physical level, the memories could come out."

"Yes! And it worked the other way, too. When I began processing the emotional trauma, my body finally started to relax."

The Body Screams

Two days after my session with Karen when the first memories of sexual molestation surfaced, I had an appointment with my physical therapist Nicole. While she worked on relaxing the muscles around my pelvis and hips, I began telling her about what I had uncovered, and my body started to unwind and shake. When she placed her hands gently over my lower abdomen, my body twitched violently, and it felt like energy was moving all the way down to my feet and out of my body.

Later that week when Iben placed her hands at my pelvic area, once again my body started unwinding and shaking. When she placed her fingers lightly on my breastbone, I writhed in pain. I had to look down because it felt like she was plunging a dagger through my heart. Intense pain and grief welled up, and I started to sob.

Afterward, I told Iben, "My body feels so much calmer, but I'm completely exhausted."

"You just went through energetic surgery," she replied.

To rid myself of my chronic physical pain over the past five years, I'd delved into my emotional and spiritual issues. Now, to deal with this huge emotional/spiritual pain, I found it extremely helpful to release the trauma at the physical level. Once again, I had a tangible experience that all aspects of my being were intertwined pieces of this healing puzzle.

The Body Knows

A month after the molestation memory surfaced, I was cleaning under my bed and found the petosky stone Father John had given me when I was nine. When I picked it up, my eyes immediately squinted shut and my pelvic floor tightened.

A few days later, I was looking for a baby picture to bring for a church activity when I came upon a picture of Father John saying Mass at my house when I was a child. There was no body reaction until I asked myself, *How do you feel?* Then, my bladder started to throb, my pelvic floor tightened, my eyes squinted shut, and I felt the familiar crinkling in my brain. I knew there was more to uncover.

About this time, I developed a curious connection with my body. If I asked my body a yes/no question related to myself, my lower spine would flex and my pelvic floor would completely relax, signifying "yes," or my pelvic floor would quickly contract and relax with an intense spasm, signifying "no."

When I told my friend Bob about this newfound capability, he laughed and said, "You don't have a gut feeling; you have a butt feeling!"

During my appointment with my physical therapist Nicole, I demonstrated my body reaction as she was working internally. I asked two questions out loud, one with an obvious "yes" response and one with an obvious "no" response. Nicole said my pelvic floor completely relaxed after the first question and then quickly spasmed in response to the second.

I told Nicole about my body's reactions when I'd discovered the picture and the stone. Then, I added, "I think new memories are starting to surface."

That night lying in bed, right before going to sleep, I wondered, *What else happened to me?* Suddenly, it occurred to me: *My body was there, and it probably knows. I can ask.* In my mind I asked, *Were you sexually molested by Father John at age* _____, filling in the blank with each year of my life. For all but three years up to age twenty-one, my body gave a clear "no" response, but at ages four, five, and nine, it responded with a huge "yes."

Next, I asked specific yes/no questions and found out that on the second night of his visit to our home when I was four, Father John sat me on his lap facing away from him and raped me. This happened again on two different nights when he visited our home when I was five and again at age nine at the church rectory.

Matching Memories

These new memories of Father John's abuse were so tough that they were difficult to believe. But when I compared them to the memories I did keep from my childhood, they matched up. With a sickened feeling, I realized that the only way Father John could have heard me asking my mother at age four about priests and pajamas was if he were standing at the end of the hall, away from his bedroom, and just out of sight.

One of my clearest memories is at age nine standing in the lobby of Father John's church and worrying about where I was going to sleep. My parents and I were traveling, and we were staying overnight at the rectory. I had always known that I'd been very sad and lonely at age nine. I remember singing the song "One Is the Loneliest Number" into the tape recorder. I also remember standing in the shower thinking there was no God and that, when I died, I would no longer exist. Such heavy thoughts for a little girl. At only nine years old, I felt utterly alone and empty. Now, I knew why I had been in such despair.

The Wolf

When I was working through feelings of betrayal, Iben said, "Father John was like a wolf in sheep's clothing."

Immediately, a memory surfaced of something that had happened six months earlier.

It was the last day of the CranioSacral course, and class was about to begin. My psychologist friend Audrey came up to me and said, "I know why we met and became practice partners. For the last two days, a clear image keeps popping into my mind, and I know it's about you. You'll have to tell me what it means, because it's a fairytale, and we didn't read them in Jamaica when I was growing up. There's a little girl in a red coat standing next to someone's bedside."

"Really?" I said. "I must be Little Red Riding Hood. And that doesn't turn out well!" Then, I explained that the little girl thinks she is bringing treats to her sick grandmother, who is actually a wolf disguised as the old lady. The wolf jumps out of the bed and devours the little girl.

Audrey replied, "Just remember, people may not be who they seem to be on the surface. Not everyone you want to be close with or to help is good for you."

"That's good advice. But the story doesn't end there. A woodsman eventually kills the wolf, and Little Red Riding Hood pops out unharmed. So, if she is really me, I'll survive and become myself again."

Believing Myself

I was already one hour late when I checked the calendar on my phone and realized I was missing a party. I drove quickly to my friend's house, and her husband, who I had never met, greeted me in the parking lot and escorted me to the condo. I apologized for being late and said I had been experiencing a lot of drama over the past week. He looked at me with a worried and questioning gaze, so I told him I was dealing with some repressed memories of sexual abuse that had recently surfaced.

Immediately, he said, "You need to be very, very careful with repressed memories. Therapists can lead you to believe they are true based on their own bias. People have been sent to jail based on memories that were completely false. But if the memories are really true, you never forget them; you can't get them out of your head."

A bit stunned, I sat down and tried to collect myself. Silently, I asked myself, *Are these sexual abuse memories real?* My lower spine immediately and forcibly flexed, and my pelvic floor relaxed—my "yes" response.

I started to appreciate that not everyone would believe me. To be honest, before my illness, I probably wouldn't have believed me, either. When my pain first began, my friend Sandy gave me the book *Expecting Adam*, written by Martha Beck. At the time, I thought that many of Beck's experiences were too far out there and unbelievable. (Now, I would accept much of what she had to say.) When I later learned that Martha had reported memories of being sexually abused by her father, I hadn't believed her. And when I heard a quote from her family that she had a very active imagination, I'd thought they were right on.

When I got home from the party, I sat down at my computer to research the validity of repressed memories online. Suddenly, my whole pelvic area tightened up. At that moment, I realized that my body-mind had given me an awareness of something I had feared and suppressed my whole life. It was time to believe my own truth.

As I was writing this section of the book, I wondered what Martha Beck had to say about her sexual abuse. So I went online and found the following explanation in a piece she'd written, called "Setting the Record Straight":

"My experience is a vivid and unshakable combination of physical evidence, memories from my childhood that never left me, new trauma memories, corroborating statements from my mother, and my looking into the work my father was undertaking at the time of the abuse that made sense of my experience. . . . I learned that lost memory is very common after traumas such as car accidents, wartime violence, criminal assault, or sexual abuse. Scientists report that young children are especially likely to repress memories of such incidents. I've come to understand that the mind can protect you until you're ready to cope with the fallout of remembering."

I went through almost the exact process as Martha did to self-validate my sexual abuse! Gaining confidence in my personal truth seemed to be a key part of this healing process.

Sometimes, I imagine telling my story to a group of people and out there in the audience is the old me. It makes me shudder! But this fear dissipates when I realize that my job is to speak my truth but never to convince anyone that it is theirs.

Healing Connections

At this point in my healing, I had developed several close connections, and this may be one of the reasons I finally felt safe enough to expose my inner truth. Following are a few examples of how my friends supported me.

The night after my session with Karen when I'd remembered the abuse, I walked across the street to my neighbor Lee's house. Just as she'd done five years earlier during the peak of my physical pain, Lee held me like a mother and dried my tears.

That week, when Alex and I were intimate, my childhood memories flashed back, and I stopped everything and started to shake and cry. This had happened the last few times we tried to be sexual together.

I said, "I'm sorry. I'm sure this will get better soon."

"You've been telling me that for twenty-five years."

In a little girl voice, I asked, "Are you mad?"

"No, just don't give the healing a timeframe. You don't know how long it will take."

"Will you stay with me?"

He replied firmly, "I'm not leaving."

When I told my friend Bob all about the memories that had surfaced, he was kind, protective, and angry at the same time. Afterward, I said, "Bob, thank you for letting me share this deep stuff." He frowned at me, shook his head, and said, "You never have to thank me."

Then, my friend Jeff and I went to the beach and spent four hours talking about everything. He stood beside me as I hammered the petosky stone into bits and threw it into the ocean. Then, he hugged me tightly.

About six months before the abuse surfaced, a choir mate of mine, Paul, and I shared our positive childhood experiences with "good guy" priests, and I told him stories about Father John. Now, I walked up to him before the church service started and said, "I lied." He listened intently to the full story, said he was sorry, and hugged me.

Paul said, "You are like one of those soldiers who goes through unspeakable things in war and finally talks about them fifty years later. Your childhood was a battle zone."

I told him how the experience had helped me grow spiritually.

"That's a good perspective," he said. "But it still sucks."

"You're right. It still sucks. As I told my therapist, it's a dramatic story; too bad it's my life."

With a sweeping motion of his arms, Paul said, "No, *this* is your life!"

Healing Little Me

The day after my body gave me such clear signals about what Father John had done to me as a child, I attended another CranioSacral session with Karen. She placed her hands lightly on my body, and I immediately felt my left-lower brain crinkling. An image of a long, red face with an elongated nose and pointy chin popped into my mind. I ignored it twice, but on its third appearance, I told Karen about it and started to cry.

I asked out loud, "Is this within me?" My body responded "no."

"Is it outside of me?" My body's answer was a clear "yes."

"Does this represent evil to me?" My body said "yes."

Suddenly, I felt like I was four, and I curled up into a ball and sobbed, soaking the sheets on the massage table. I was so scared. I tried to scream, and Father John clamped his hand over my mouth and continued to hurt me. He said that if I told anyone he would not love me anymore and my mother would not love me, either.

Karen asked, "What does this little girl need in order to heal?"

I replied without hesitation. "She needs to be adored, caressed, and accepted."

"Can you do that for her now?"

In my mind, I held myself tight and kissed my little face all over. Then, I had a clear image of my four-year-old self throwing herself on the ground and having a tantrum. As the adult, I placed my hand on her back and told her, "You have every right to be mad. It is okay to let it out. I love you very much."

After about five minutes, I asked myself, "Have you had enough time? Can I move to age five?" My spine flexed, and my pelvic floor relaxed—my "yes" response.

Immediately, my calves and buttocks went into a spasm, and I felt like I was five years old again. I was seated on Father John's lap in my nightgown, and I knew what was going to happen. I was trying to brace myself for the attack. I was really angry but too afraid to show it.

Karen asked, "Could you help yourself release the tension in your body?"

So I envisioned me as an adult massaging the calves and rear of my little-girl self. Then, I had a clear image of five-year-old me running around my childhood bedroom and frantically destroying the place. The adult me looked upon her with understanding, acceptance, and love.

After a few minutes, I asked myself, "Is it okay if I move to age nine?" My body response was "yes." Then, in my mind I heard my younger selves saying, "Go, go. She is really hurting and needs the most help."

Suddenly, I felt like I was nine again, confused, and despairing. Father John told me I had brought this on myself, and I felt sexual and bad. As this memory surfaced, I felt my whole left side, from my calf to my hip, tighten up on Karen's massage table.

I said, "This is when I shut down the emotional, sexual, and spiritual sides of me. It was not safe, and I needed to protect myself. It literally feels like these parts of me ascended up and away."

"Could you ask your younger selves if they are ready to accept these parts of you again?" Karen asked.

I told Karen, "I've let the spiritual, feminine, and emotional sides back in over the past years, but not the sexual side."

I encouraged myself to let the sexual part of me come in, and it started to feel like my pelvic area, near my bladder, was filling up. This was interesting to me because this was the area of my pain and of the second chakra, which represents sexual expression. Suddenly, it stopped filling up, and I had a keen sense that the vessel was really beaten up and partly broken.

I told myself, "There is no hurry. Take all the time you need. It can trickle in over time."

I had no idea I was so shut down in the sexual area until my sexuality began making an appearance. In the beginning when the sexual part of me was opening up, my automatic fear response would surface, and I would feel my calf and butt muscles tighten and the familiar crinkling in my brain. Then, I would have to stop and calm my body and mind. Gradually, over time, I started to let the sexual part of myself live.

As the session with Karen was coming to a close, I asked her if other people dialogued with past selves.

"All the time," she said.

Karen explained that Dr. Upledger, the founder of the CranioSacral approach, did this type of work with patients intuitively, and it was effective. Now, brain-imaging studies show that thinking about or imagining an event activates the same areas of the brain as when the event actually happens. Karen added that, in her experience, patients can revisit the past like I did and use this process to change their body's response to the trauma.

Karen also told me that, during our session, the "yes" and "no" body responses I'd demonstrated consistently matched the craniosacral rhythms she felt throughout my body. She encouraged me to continue this inner dialogue.

Hearing My Truth

Iben asked me to write a letter to Father John to get out all my emotions. She encouraged me, saying, "It is your birthright to feel however you want to feel. Embrace it; make it raw. Know that these emotions have been infesting your body for almost fifty years."

When I sat down in front of my computer to write my letter to Father John, I asked myself, *How did you feel when this happened at age four?* Very clear sentences popped into my mind, most of them followed by my body's spontaneous and firm "yes" response. Whenever this happened, I took it as a sign that the thought was my inner truth and wrote it down. I repeated this process for all three ages I'd experienced the sexual abuse.

Following are the inner truths that came to me that day:

Age Four

I feel so small and helpless around you.

I see your face changing, and I'm scared.

It feels like you are ripping me apart.

I tell you it hurts, and you keep doing it.

I thought you loved me, and I don't know why you are hurting me.

I start to cry out in pain, and you cover my mouth and hurt me even more down there.

I am mad that you don't talk to me or look at me.

I am scared you are coming back. I am looking at the door and hoping it doesn't open.

I feel thrown away.

Age Five

I think my mom said it was okay for Fr. John to use my body.

I don't think my mother loves me.

No one listens to me.

No one cares about me.

I am all alone.

If I cry out, I will be hurt.

I can't control what happens to me.

I am afraid of his part down there.

Age Nine

I brought this on myself.

I made him want me.

I am too needy and clingy.

I am a problem, a burden.

No one loves me.

I want to die.

I hate sex.

I hate the sexual part of men.

There is no God.

When I reviewed this list with Iben, she remarked at how clearly it showed how the same trauma affected me differently at various ages. At age four, I'd felt confusion, pain, and fear. At age five, I'd felt abandoned, especially by my mother. At age nine, I'd appreciated the sexual nature of the act and blamed myself; I'd lost my faith and felt despair.

Eventually, I wrote my angry letter to Father John and read all of it to Iben. As I was speaking, she quietly put my feelings into a broader perspective, saying things like, "You are feeling the injustice of it all." "You feel like a victim." "Now, you are feeling superior."

Eventually, I rewrote each sentence of the letter so that it began with "I." This enabled me to own my emotions and to feel more in charge and less like a victim.

Iben helped me to appreciate how this experience had affected me. I realized that I hadn't felt safe with the priest who was God's messenger or with my parents. There was nowhere to turn. Internally, I was angry, and I felt unworthy, separate, and abandoned. To alleviate those feelings, I frantically tried to be perfect and to connect with others.

Reaction and Suffering

One Sunday before church, Bob told me about how his father, who was a good provider but emotionally distant, occasionally punished him with the whip he used on the dogs. As a result of that experience, Bob had adopted the attitude that no one would ever bring him down. We talked about how that trauma had molded his personality and future experiences.

I told him I'd had a similar thought about my sexual abuse. It was not the physical act itself but the reactions in my heart and mind that had dictated how the experience affected my life.

Bob agreed and said that each of his brothers had a different reaction to their father's emotional distance and physical punishments. The first brother had driven himself for achievement; the second brother had become sensitive and broken; and Bob had decided to be lighthearted and pretend like it had not affected him. We agreed that the same trauma affects everyone differently, based on their make-up and their response to the experience.

Over time, I realized that my response to my sexual abuse subconsciously altered my filters and changed how I perceived myself and my world. That response then influenced the dynamics I created in my life. My internal reaction to this trauma became the root of my belief system and the common dynamics of my behavior.

Following are the subsequent reactions that played out in my relationships and experiences throughout my life:

Shock: I couldn't understand how someone who had been kind to me had also hurt me.

Fear: I didn't feel safe at a basic level.

Victim: I felt inferior, abandoned, and unlovable.

Anger: I bristled at the injustice of it all and suppressed this rage.

Superiority: I felt better than all the people who had let me down.

I don't blame myself for any of these reactions. I was doing my best to feel safe and survive, and I couldn't consciously choose how the situation affected me. But understanding that my response to the trauma had prolonged my pain put me firmly back in control. I couldn't change what had happened to me, but I could change the fearful beliefs that I'd adopted and were so limiting. I knew this was the healing path.

I remembered something Iben once said. "How you perceive the situation makes the experience. That is your reality."

Seeing the Light

When the memories of being raped throughout my childhood surfaced, I told Bob about them.

He said, "Look at what you've been able to experience."

"You're right. I really have experienced depths of despair and peaks of joy. If we are here to experience all of life, this trauma helped me do it."

"Yes, and in that way, it was a gift."

"Iben, my life coach, told me something that fits here. She said it's hard to appreciate the flame of a candle when you are holding it in front of the sun, but against a dark background, the light is obvious."

Back to Church

In September of 2012, I stepped into a local Catholic church and sat in the front pew, right in front of the life-sized crucifix. Just like I'd planned, I silently made the following declaration: *I accept everything Jesus was about: love, compassion, acceptance, and healing. But I completely reject the man-made part of this religion: the power, hierarchy, dogma, and fear.*

As I stood to leave, I noticed the sacristy, altar, and stained-glass windows—similar to the ones that had been a familiar backdrop to countless life memories—and sat back down. I realized that within these walls, of both this church and the church of my childhood, I had experienced more than just oppression and fear. I had also felt connection and love.

Shutting my eyes, I envisioned the constricting thoughts and feelings I had about my experiences with the church as a thick, black sweater enveloping me and then slipping the heavy, dark sweater off my shoulders and laying it on the seat behind me. I felt some of the weight lift off me, but I knew I was carrying more. So I placed my hands on different parts of my body as I pictured whatever dark emotion related to my interactions with the church might reside there and then imagined it being cleared away. After about a half hour, I thought of myself as a transparent vessel and then envisioned that open space being filled with healing white light.

Just then, a little girl of about four years old bounded into the church with her mother, bubbling with questions and excited chatter.

"Shhhh," her mother said. "You have to be quiet. You'll bother that lady who is praying."

I turned around and said, "Please, let her talk. I don't mind. In fact, I like it." It felt a bit like I was giving my four-year-old self permission to speak and to be herself within this sanctuary.

After they left, I picked up the book of hymns and asked myself if I should open it randomly. My lower back immediately flexed, and my pelvic floor relaxed—my body's "yes" response. I asked three times, and each time my body responded in the same way. Every time I opened the book, the song had special meaning for me. The first song was "We Are the Light of the World," and the phrase, "We are the light of the world /

May our light shine before all," popped off the page and into my heart. The second song was "Take My Hands," and the words, "Take my hands / they speak now for my heart / and by their actions they will show their love," seemed to be written for me. Throughout my life, both as a physical therapist and then with the new energy work, using my hands has always felt fulfilling and healing for me. The third hymn I opened to was "On Eagle's Wings"—my mother's favorite song. The last time I'd heard it was five years before, when my pain was at its peak. Sitting in this same church and singing this same hymn had triggered my first emotional release at the very beginning of my healing journey.

When I asked if I should open the music issue again, my pelvic floor quickly spasmed, which I now equate with a "no" response.

Next, I asked if I should randomly open the book containing the order of the Mass and some Psalms, and twice I received my body's "yes" response. The first reading didn't mean anything in particular to me, but the second reading spoke about how suffering can lead to wisdom.

As I was leaving the church, the janitor stopped me and said, "I watched you praying today. You were truly in the presence of God." Then, he told me many stories of faith and healing from his own life and how he had been completely cured from end-stage, metastatic cancer. He said he cleaned the church and provided support for those with cancer in thanks for the gift of his life.

As I headed to my car in the bright sunshine, I realized that the bladder pain I'd felt when I'd entered the church was now gone. In its place was overwhelming gratitude for this healing day.

Really? Gratitude?

After Iben and I had worked through the sexual abuse for several months, she encouraged me to write another letter using the following prompt: "Thank you, Father John, for abusing me, because I have learned this, and this, and this about myself, and it has allowed me to expand." She told me not to just write a list of how I'd managed or survived the abuse but to describe how the experience had helped me grow on a soul level. She encouraged me to take my time, not push myself, and make sure it was genuine.

Here are a few examples from my list:

- *I experienced a distinct contrast between being disconnected and connected to my own spirit.*
- *I developed empathy for others who feel less-than and are in despair.*
- *I learned to love myself at a very deep level.*
- *I experienced a wide range of human emotions, from the depths of despair to absolute joy.*
- *I know how it feels to live with hierarchy, domination, fear, and control and to consciously choose love, acceptance, and healing.*

If I were to condense my angry letter, about ten main feelings would be repeated over and over. But my thank-you letter contained thirty-two distinct points of gratitude! Sometimes, when the challenge is great, the potential for growth is great, too.

Iben said that when we grow into gratitude and allow ourselves to feel it in the heart, we transmute the experience. She said that this was a body process, and when I could revisit the abuse mentally and not have a reaction in my body, I would know that I had moved past it. She told me that I was healing a full dynamic of dominance and hierarchy, and soon I wouldn't need to experience it anymore. She said that when I felt equal, I would feel compassion for everyone in the dynamic.

Iben was right. As I healed from the abuse, the reaction I'd had to hierarchy throughout my life dissipated, and my internal agitation was often replaced with compassion.

15

The Journey Is Everything

Three of my caregivers—my physical therapist, Julie; my acupuncturist, Pam; and my urogynecologist, Dr. Noblett—gave a seminar on the multidisciplinary treatment for pelvic pain and used my case as an example. Inspired by a sign in one of the treatment rooms at the Healing Sanctuary, Julie had included the phrase "The Journey Is Everything" on her concluding slide.

Two years earlier, I'd asked Pam where she'd bought the sign and then purchased one for myself. It has been hanging over my bed ever since. From opposite sides of the treatment table, both my caregivers and I have witnessed the path through pain. We've seen the strong connections between the body, mind, and spirit, and we've observed the instructive potential of this rough journey.

When my pain levels were high, I often asked my caregivers if they thought I'd be pain-free and when they thought it would happen. As a caregiver, I knew they didn't have the answers, but as a patient, I had to ask, anyway.

In response, Pam would always say that life is never perfect. None of us would ever be pain-free, and there would always be challenges in life. She would remind me that to have no challenges was to be dead. I always conceded her point but then added that I was really, really ready for this particular challenge to pass. In the beginning, Pam and I had different perspectives on this trip I was taking, and both were valid. For me, it was a journey through pelvic pain, and my destination was a place where I was pain-free. For Pam, it was the larger journey through life, and my pelvic pain was just one leg of the trip. Over time, as the pain diminished, I could see the journey from her broader perspective.

Before my pain began, I'd walked through my life looking up the road to a future destination—the perfect life. The qualities of this life would often change, but what stayed constant was my discontent when my present circumstances fell short of this ideal.

Then, through these painful years, my perspective shifted, and I often focused on walking itself and on experiencing the varied scenery and terrain all around me. I started to accept that sometimes the journey would be easy, beautiful, and fun, and sometimes it would be difficult, ugly, and painful. My life didn't need to be perfect in order to be valuable, true, and right. When I let go of the expectations and control, life became more of an adventure.

Walking in this dark place also forced me to use other senses to figure out where I was going. Before my illness, I listened only to my mind to define my world and guide my life. But now, my body gives me information and a peaceful intuition often chimes in, speaking the truth of my spirit. I will continue walking on my life's journey, with all its inevitable peaks and valleys. But on the rest of my trip, my body, mind, and spirit will all have a voice.

Recently, my friend Christine, who survived stage-three breast cancer, reminded me that you never "arrive" and you are never perfectly healed on all levels. She said that the meaning is in the process, in the journey itself.

Inner Truth

There is an old folder on my computer that I created before my illness, called "Inspirational Writing." Before my pain began, I rarely wrote beyond my professional duties, so the folder contained only three documents: the memories of my mother's last days, the writing about Father John, and a description of my marriage. In each, I describe the relationship in a positive, bigger-than-life way. Now, I knew that these were the main protective stories of my life, and in order to heal, I had to unravel them and appreciate my truth.

Over the years of healing, I read through my old writings, revisited my most vivid memories, uncovered my core beliefs, felt my buried emotions, and listened to my body. In time, I started to realize that what I was uncovering was not new. It seemed like I held knowledge about the reasons for my pain and the path for healing at many levels. Healing was the process of becoming more and more aware of this inner truth.

Discovering Myself

Prior to my illness, I could have been described as compassionate, busy, competent, and driven. What I didn't know was that I felt fearful and unsafe at a basic level. I was on high alert and looking for signs that I was loved. I knew I had a big loving capacity, but I wanted it to flow back to me to fill me up. When it didn't, I held anger and resentment.

I started this journey to get out of physical pain, and ended up becoming more aware of all these aspects of myself. I looked honestly at the parts of me I had ignored for a lifetime: my full body, my darker sides, my emotions, my feminine side, and my spirituality. I uncovered the sexual trauma and the patterns in my thinking and behavior that had grown out of this experience and affected my life. Over time, I started to understand, accept, and love myself. And when I felt more secure with myself, my body began to relax.

About five years ago, at the end of my first session with my psychologist, Jackie, she asked, "Do you need to be perfect in order to be loved?" I wasn't sure then, but now I know that I am loved and accepted just for who I am by other people and, most important, by myself.

At my mother's funeral, an aunt I had seen only a handful of times in my life tapped me on the shoulder and said, "When you were about three, you came up to me, smiled, and said, 'You're going to love me.'" In many ways, that joyful, confident, and impish me now shines forth again.

A Changed Life

As I healed inside, my life changed for the better.

Before my pain began, there was a clear hierarchy in my marriage and in our home. Now, there is much more connection, equality, and compassion between us, and I know that my healing was integral to making this change.

Before my illness, I felt isolated and lonely, and I was never comfortable with women. Now, I have very close friends who are old and young and from all walks of life, and many of them are women.

My work now clearly reflects the authentic me. I still write, but the content has changed from technical lectures to stories about the mind, body, and spirit. I still work with people in pain, but now I have a more holistic view of health. I used to just work, work, work, but now I also play.

One day after updating Iben on how I was doing and what was going on with me, I smiled and said, "Can you believe this is *my* life?"

Chronic Pain: The Ultimate Spiritual Teacher

During my first bout of pelvic pain, my acupuncturist, Pam, told me that I could use my pelvic pain as a messenger to give me information about when I was a bit dissociated from my true self. In this way, the pain was actually a gift. Truly, when I'm in pain, it never *feels* like a gift! But Pam was right. The pain forced me to look at what I'm doing, thinking, feeling, and carrying, because those mental and emotional issues were wrapped up in the discomfort.

The pain was the ultimate spiritual teacher because it told me clearly when something caused me stress or fear. Then, it motivated me to take a more expanding, loving path, so I could be physically comfortable. I would never have worked so diligently on my emotional/spiritual health if my body hadn't pushed me. Nothing is a better motivator than getting out of pain!

I summed up this healing experience in my journal:

I was well acquainted with who I had become, but over time I met who had started the journey. As I picked up the layers of characteristics I had donned to be safe and survive, I glimpsed the unchanging nature of my soul.

Spiritual Transformation

My friend Jeff told me that in many accounts of spiritual transformation, the person ends up floating around in a beautiful, peaceful state. Not me. Just when I think I've arrived, my humanness rises up to kick me in the butt (often, literally)! The difference is that I can now see my part in the dynamics I'm experiencing, and I usually see when old patterns are sneaking up on me and causing me to suffer. Sometimes, this insight comes after I have acted, and I find myself humbly apologizing. Surprisingly, when I am vulnerable and honest, other people often respond in kind. For me, transformation is a process of growing in awareness rather than achieving a certain state of being or arriving at a perfect destination.

Iben once told me that being spiritual was not about being otherworldly, devoid of emotion, and above it all. Rather, it is about being fully present in your body and in your life. Instead, it is no longer feeling a separation between the body, the world around you, and universal energy. It is having a connection with God (or the Universe, or All One) and with others in this shared human experience. Over the years, I have experienced the truth of Iben's words at deeper and deeper levels.

When I first met Pam, she recommended the book *The Path of Transformation*, by Shakti Gawain. Recently, I came across it again and decided to read it. In this book, written more than twenty years ago, the author describes the classic steps of spiritual transformation: a healing crisis, a spiritual awakening, mental healing, deep emotional work, physical healing, and moving out into the world. She laid out exactly what had happened on my journey. Once again, I recognized that my process of healing through the layers wasn't unique.

Then, a thought immediately surfaced: *Wait a minute! I thought I was unique and special! Is there nothing sacred?*

But another thought quickly rose up: *Perhaps the fact that your experience is not unique means it **is** sacred.*

The Healing Power of Imperfection

Five years after my illness emerged, I found a poem I'd written at eighteen years old that spoke about perfection.

Revealing experiences lead me to pause and inspect myself arrayed in a picture frame.
Shocked by self-knowledge I intently analyze the painter's work.
Bright yellow and sorrow blue blend.
Rich deepness in stormy calmness
Browsers recognize the picture's uniqueness.
Only with insight can they see the fine flaw lines.
Capable of perfection the painter never abolished weakness.
Has the painter placed the fine flaws for interest sake?
Or is the mistake a building block for self-knowledge?

Now, thirty-two years after writing that poem, I can answer the question at the end with a resounding "Yes!" Over the years, it was this struggle with the imperfection of my body, my flaws, and my weaknesses that led to greater self-knowledge and healing.

As these ideas were percolating, someone emailed me a poem by Leonard Cohen that clearly reinforced this message.

Ring the bells that still can ring.
Forget your perfect offering.
There is a crack, a crack in everything.
That's how the light gets in.

Curing versus Healing

The first book I read when the pain began was *Love and Survival,* by the cardiologist Dr. Dean Ornish. One passage jumped out at me then and seems to summarize my experience even today:

"Curing is when the physical disease gets measurably better. Healing is a process of becoming whole. Even the words heal, whole, and holy come from the same root. . . . In the process of healing, you reach a place of wholeness and deep inner peace from which you can deal with illness with much less fear and suffering and much greater clarity and compassion. While curing is wonderful when it occurs, healing is often more meaningful because it takes you to a place of greater freedom from suffering."

During my journey with pain, I experienced both curing and healing. The physical disease got better, and I am currently pain-free. But more important, this rough road healed me. Now, I am often joyful—for no real reason and for every real reason.

And now, almost five and a half years after my illness began, I can clearly see that my pain was the catalyst and healing is the story.

Treatments for Chronic Pelvic Pain

When my pain levels were high, reading through a book was difficult and sometimes impossible. I had one question I wanted answered: "How can I decrease this pain?" If you are at that point in your healing, this section is for you. It lists all the treatments I undertook to heal my pain, which are described in greater detail throughout the book.

If you are despairing at the length of this list, keep in mind that the process I went through to heal my body is unique to me. There are many different medical issues and treatments for chronic pelvic pain, and the combination of these will be different for every person. I am sharing my experiences to give you ideas to consider, options to try, and things to discuss with your caregivers. If you are in pain, I hope my experience gives you information that you can use to develop your individual healing plan.

Bladder Pain and Inflammation
- Medications
  - Elmiron®: Orally administered heparin to coat the inner lining of the bladder
- Diet/Supplements
  - Chinese herbs
  - Pre-Relief®: Over-the-counter medication taken prior to eating acidic foods
  - Low acid IC diet: To decrease irritation of inner walls of the bladder
  - Anti-inflammatory diet

- Instillations: Medication placed into bladder with a catheter
  - DMSO (dimethyl sulfoxide): An older, traditional medication for IC
  - Heparin: In combination with a steroid and anesthetic
- Physical Therapy Modalities
  - Microcurrent electrical stimulation
  - Cold laser
- Bladder Pain Relievers
  - Pyridium® or Urelle®: Prescription medications taken orally; bladder anesthetics
  - Transcutaneous electrical nerve stimulation (TENS)
  - Heating pad or Thermacare® warm pack: Placed over the lower abdomen
  - Warm bath or whirlpool

Pelvic Floor Myopathy/Myalgia

- Physical therapy
- Massage therapy
- Home program: Internal and external pelvic muscle work
- Warm or hot whirlpool
- Paradoxical relaxation meditation
- Deep diaphragmatic breathing
- Hatha yoga, especially long-held poses that stretch the low back, hip, and pelvic area (i.e., yin yoga)
- Baclofen® or Valium® suppositories
- Trigger point injections of anesthetic (Marcaine® and lidocaine)

Neurological Ramp-Up and Emotions

- Cymbalta®
- Aerobic exercise to help get the circulation and endorphins moving
- Yoga
- Meditation
- Acupuncture
- Psychotherapy
- Reiki/energy work
- Multi-dimensional life coaching
- Myofascial Release treatment
- CranioSacral treatment

APPENDIX 2

Pain Management Strategies

This appendix includes the details of how I communicated with my caregivers during my illness and how I organized my plan of action. This information is presented not as a prescription but as an example to consider.

Writing a Medical History

Here are the main points I included in my personal medical history:

- Significant past medical history not related to pelvic pain
- The diagnosis of pelvic pain, including when my symptoms began, what these symptoms were, and the diagnostic tests performed
- Description of the current levels of pain (see the section of this appendix titled "Describing Pain") and how the pain levels changed over time
- List of other symptoms. Of course, these will vary from person to person. Mine included urinary frequency and urgency, fecal urgency and dumping, and fatigue.
- How the condition impacted my life, such as sleep, basic needs, daily tasks, work, and recreation
- Treatments tried and current treatments
- Medications tried and current medications

To each follow-up visit with a caregiver, I brought notes on how my pain, symptoms, and activity status had changed since the last visit. I also wrote down any new instructions they gave me. That way, I didn't have the pressure of remembering everything. After all, life was stressful enough!

Describing Pain

To describe my pain to caregivers, I would specify the following:

- Pain Rating: 0–10 scale, using the following descriptors as a guide

0	No pain
2	Mild pain: can be ignored
4	Moderate pain: interferes with tasks
6	Moderate pain: interferes with concentration
8	Severe pain: interferes with basic needs
10	Worst pain possible: bed rest required

- Location: Using words and/or pointing to the area
- Type of Pain: For example, dull ache, sharp/shooting pain, or burning sensation
- Percent of the Day: The percent of my waking time that I was in pain

Here is an example of how I would have described my bladder pain in the sixth month of my illness:

The pain is centered right above my pubic bone. It is a throbbing, nerve pain accompanied by the feeling that my bladder is extremely full and someone is sitting on my stomach. It is a level 4, and it bothers me on average about 40% of the day.

Charting Pain

On pages 252–253 are two sets of charts describing my pain: one set for January 2008 (six months into my condition) and another set for January 2009. Each set contains two charts: a spreadsheet and a graph. Each spreadsheet includes three sections: (1) Symptoms, (2) Treatments, and (3) Daily Management. The Symptoms section specifies both the pain-level rating and the percentage of the day the pain persisted, and this data is displayed in the corresponding graph.

JANUARY 2008

	T 1	W 2	Th 3	F 4	S 5	Su 6	M 7	T 8	W 9	Th 10	F 11	S 12	Su 13	M 14
Symptoms														
Bladder Pain	3	3	3	3	4	5	4	4	4	4	4	3	3	4
Bladder % of Day	2	1	1	0.5	6	7	5	5	4	4	4	1	1	5
Menstrual Cycle												*	*	*
Treatments														
Suppositories							*	*	*	*	*			
Instillation										*				
Physical Therapy				*			*			*	*			
Psychotherapy		*							*					
Yoga				*						*			*	
Acupuncture								*						
Daily Management														
Elmiron BID	*	*	*	*	*	*	*	*	*	*	*	*	*	*
Cymbalta 60 mg QD	*	*	*	*	*	*	*	*	*	*	*	*	*	*
Home Program	*	*	*	*	*	*			*	*	*	*	*	*
Cardio Exercise	*		*				*	*		*		*		
Core Strengthening	*		*						*		*			
Meditation	*								*					

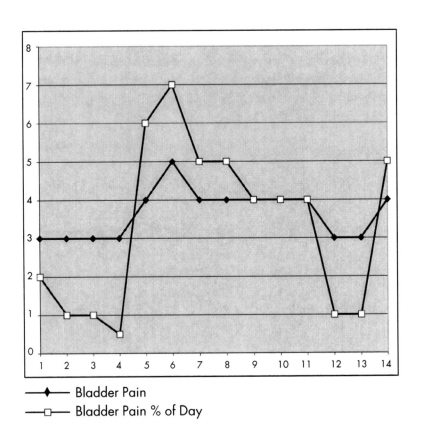

Bladder Pain

Bladder Pain % of Day

JANUARY 2009

	Th 1	F 2	S 3	Su 4	M 5	T 6	W 7	Th 8	F 9	S 10	Su 11	M 12	T 13	W 14
Symptons														
Bladder Pain	3	3	0	0	3	3	0	0	0	0	0	0	0	0
Bladder % of Day	1	4	0	0	3	1	0	0	0	0	0	0	0	0
Menstrual Cycle														
Stress		*			*	*	*	*	*					
GI Symptoms		G		D	C		D							
Treatments														
Suppositories		*	*											
Instillation		*												
Physical Therapy								*						*
Psychotherapy														
Yoga				*						*			*	
Acupuncture	*						*							
Massage Therapy														
Daily Management														
Cymbalta 30 mg QD	*	*	*	*	*	*	*	*	*	*	*	*	*	*
Home Program	*	*	*	*	*	*	*		*	*	*	*	*	
Cardio Exercise				*	*	*						*		
Core Strenghening				*	*							*		
Meditation			*	*	*	*	*							

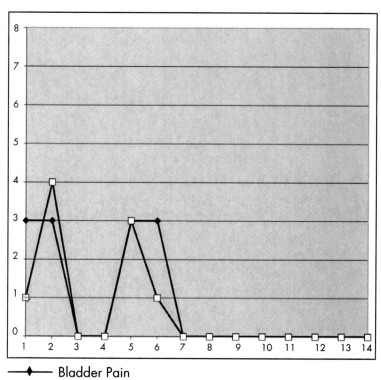

Bladder Pain

Bladder Pain % of Day

My spreadsheet and graph were invaluable tools for seeing the general trend of my condition, because my progress was slow and tended to wax and wane. It was unclear how I was doing day to day or even week to week, but when I looked at my status over the months or years, my progress was obvious. For example, when my spreadsheets and graphs from January of 2008 and 2009 are compared, the level of bladder pain and the percentage of the day I was experiencing the pain had both decreased. The improvement in my condition was also reflected in my interventions. I no longer took the medication Elmiron, and the dosage of my pain medication Cymbalta was cut in half. In addition, although my treatments were the same, the frequency of my visits had decreased.

It is important to chart the symptom(s) that impact your life the most and that change over time. For example, my bladder pain was the most annoying and life-altering symptom of all. What fluctuated the most was not the level of pain but the percentage of the day it bothered me.

Tracking both the average level of pain (1–10) and the percentage of the day you are in pain (1 = 10% of the day and 10 = 100% of the day) can capture your pain experience for the day.

If you have more than one area of pain, it is wise to chart them separately. I kept track of my two main areas of pain—the bladder and pelvic-floor muscles—as well as my urinary frequency. For clarity, these example spreadsheets and graphs show only the data related to the bladder.

Include other symptoms (beyond pain) if they are bothersome. For example, initially, I recorded how often I urinated during a 24-hour period because urinary frequency is a common symptom of BPS/IC. On my chart, 4 indicated the typical number of voidings over a 24-hour period (usually, once a night and every three to four hours during the day), and any number above 4 indicated I was voiding more frequently.

Consider tracking other physical issues to see if they are a factor related to your pain. For example, I kept track of the days of my menstrual cycle to see whether my pain cycled with these monthly body changes.

The treatments section allowed me to keep track of which therapies I attended on a specific day. I could then look at my pain levels for that day or the next day to see whether there was a trend. This gave me information about whether certain treatments were effective in decreasing my pain.

The daily management section allowed me to see whether my medications and self-treatment activities corresponded to a decrease in pain over time. In addition, this was a reminder to keep up with my home program.

As the condition changes over time, it is important to modify the factors that are recorded on the spreadsheet. For example, several changes were made in my second year spreadsheet. I began seeing a massage therapist, and kept track of these visits. I also began to chart my stress levels and my gastrointestinal symptoms more closely, using the symbols G (gas), D (diarrhea), and C (constipation).

If the level of detail in my charts is overwhelming, you can simplify yours. The main thing to include in your chart is the level (1–10) of the physical symptom(s) that affects your life the most and changes over time. In addition, mark the dates when treatments are started or stopped. Keep in mind that a chart doesn't need to be complicated or made on a computer to capture valuable information about your condition and to effectively communicate your experience with your caregivers.

Sample Action Plan

Here is an action plan I created about six months into my pain.

Daily Tasks	Flare-Up Options		Future Options
	Bladder	Pelvic Floor	
Take Medications	Instillation	Baclofen	CranioSacral therapy
Internal Trigger Points	IC Diet	Physical Therapy	Myofascial Release
External Myofascial Work	PreRelief	Whirlpool	Acupuncture
Foam Roller Exercises	Whirlpool		
Cardio Exercise	TENS		
Core Strengthening			
Meditation			
Chart Daily